I Believe in Evan

I Believe in Evan

MY FIGHT TO SAVE MY BABY FROM A DEVASTATING BRAIN INJURY AND THE FORCES AGAINST US

ELISE SCHWARZ

JOHN BLAKE

Published by John Blake Publishing Ltd,
3 Bramber Court, 2 Bramber Road,
London W14 9PB, England

www.johnblakebooks.com

www.facebook.com/johnblakebooks 🄵
twitter.com/jblakebooks 🄴

This edition published in 2016

ISBN: 978 1 78418 980 8

British Library Cataloguing-in-Publication Data:

A catalogue record for this book is available from the British Library.

Design by www.envydesign.co.uk

Printed in Great Britain by CPL Group (UK) Ltd

©

The right of Elise Sch
asserted by her in accor

Papers used by John Bla
wood grown in sustaina
environm

Every attempt has been
were unobtainable. We would be grateful if the appropriate people could contact us.

Contents

Part One

Our Beginnings

Sitting at my desk on the forty-first-floor, I stare out of the window at the January sun glancing off the snow on the Manhattan streets below. I am suspended between thoughts of work and home. My phone rings. 'This is Elise,' I answer. I instantly recognise the screams of my four-and-a-half-month-old baby boy, Evan. Then I hear the babysitter. She is hysterical.

'Norma, calm down and tell me what's happening,' I say, my own voice breaking.

After a few more tries, I can finally make out her saying, 'There's something wrong with Evan. He's turning blue.'

'Call an ambulance!' I scream down the line.

More hysteria from the other end of the phone. I can still hear Evan crying.

'Okay, I'll call it!' I shout, over the noise, and hang up on her.
Dialling 911, I can hardly believe what is happening.

'My baby boy is turning blue,' I say, as clearly as possible to
the dispatcher.

I give her all the details she asks for and tell her I will be at the
apartment too, as soon as I can get there.

Grabbing my coat and bag I run to the elevator, take it to the
ground floor, then run out of the building and down into the
subway, where a train is just pulling in. I jump on board and it
takes me all the way to the 72nd Street stop without any delay.
The entire time I pray and pray Evan will be okay.

Pushing past people to get to the top of the station stairs,
I run out into the cold air and see the ambulance outside my
building. The traffic miraculously stops just when I need it to
and as I run across the street I see the paramedics wheel out
a stretcher.

Norma is sitting on it, holding Evan.

'It's okay, everything is okay!' shouts one of the paramedics,
holding up a hand to me. I run to Evan. He looks so pale that
the little strip of blond hair on the top of his head stands out
darkly against his skin. As we all clamber into the ambulance,
the paramedic explains that when they arrived Evan was
breathing normally, but they are taking him to the emergency
room to have him checked out anyway. I am beside myself
with relief. I want to hold Evan tight to me, but that means
switching seats with Norma, and I don't want to waste any
time getting to the hospital.

The paramedics take us to Cornell University Hospital on the

Our Beginnings

Upper East Side. I don't get to hold Evan until after he has been admitted, but when I do I give him the longest hug, fighting tears, and tell him over and over again how much I love him. He looks perfectly fine by now. We get ourselves settled in one of the bays and Norma tries to explain what has happened. Evan had woken from a nap, started crying, and then started turning blue. She was worried that he had stopped breathing. She says she called me first and then she tried CPR. She shows me how. I have never seen CPR performed on a baby and am grateful that she knows how to do it as I certainly don't. After an hour or so, I tell Norma she can go home, thanking her profusely. She starts crying. It has been a trying experience for her, too.

Doctors and nurses come and go in a steady flow. They ask me all sorts of questions about Evan and our life together. I try to give them as much detail as I can. I'm a single mother by choice. Evan and I live in a small studio apartment on the Upper West Side. I was at work and didn't see what happened. Norma, his babysitter, had been with him all day. Nothing like this has happened before, he is a perfect baby. Seizures? There is some history in my family. I don't know about Evan's father. I used donor sperm and there wasn't anything about the donor's medical history that rang any alarm bells. Evan gets a bit colicky, and cries a bit, but babies do, don't they? They have spoken to Norma at length, too.

Evan and I spend the next forty-eight hours in a room in the paediatric wing, with three other babies, each with their parents at the bedside. I don't have family in New York. My mother is still in Scotland, where I'm from, and my dad died a few months

3

ago. I have lots of friends in New York, but I don't call anyone to let them know we are in hospital. It doesn't occur to me. I am focused on Evan and on what is happening. When the extended families of the other babies come to visit, I feel a little sad, and very alone.

After a range of tests, including chest X-rays, blood tests and constant monitoring, the doctors still have no idea what has happened to cause Evan to turn blue. There has been no recurrence since we've been admitted, and they have started to lose the air of concern they had when we first arrived. In the early afternoon of the third day, two student doctors stop by and one of them, a tall female doctor with a heavy jaw and dark-rimmed glasses, says, 'We're going to get neurology involved. We don't think there's anything going on there, but if there was – if he had a knock or something – and we let him go home without discovering it, it would be a bad miss.'

I am concerned, of course, but I put my full faith in these doctors. Why shouldn't I? Within the hour, Evan and I are taken down the hall to another department, where a technician performs an ultrasound. It's a very simple procedure. He runs a plastic wand over the surface of Evan's head, and a grainy black and white image appears on the screen.

'I still have to make a report of this,' he says, 'but I can tell you right now I don't see anything wrong here at all.'

Evan and I go back to our shared room, and a little while later the heavy-jawed doctor comes back in and tells us everything was fine, and that Evan has been given the all-clear by the attending doctor.

Our Beginnings

'It's being diagnosed as an ALTE,' she explains. An 'Apparent Life Threatening Event'. That's all. We can go home.

Delighted and relieved, I wheel Evan out of the hospital in his buggy. We walk all the way home, across town, through the park, along our street where the ambulance had been just a couple of days before, and up and into our cosy little apartment as quickly as we can. I take him out of his stroller and hold his warm body tight as I weep into the furry orange hood of his blue dinosaur snowsuit.

We spend the next three days at home. It's the weekend, and Norma isn't due back until Tuesday. I spend these three days slowly processing what has happened. I call my mum in Scotland. I had talked to her a lot from the hospital and kept her abreast of what was going on.

The only news from her end is that a silver birch in the front garden of the family home has had to be cut down. It was damaged a few months before in a storm that felled its parent, a much larger and formidable tree that had stood in our front garden for a hundred years or so. I feel a certain upset that this second tree has come down. Then I feel annoyance and irritability about even thinking about a stupid tree amid the worry of the past few days.

We have a regular appointment with Evan's paediatrician scheduled on the Sunday. 'An ALTE means they have no idea,' our doctor says, in his usual dry tone. He checks Evan over, reassures me he is fine, and then sends us home.

Tuesday comes, and with it Norma. When she arrives, I thank her all over again for having reacted to the situation, particularly for having the presence of mind to perform CPR on Evan. We have a long conversation. I tell her that it had been really difficult for me to understand her on the phone; she hadn't remained calm, but also she had used her mobile phone, and reception wasn't great in my apartment. I tell her I will pick up a land phone on the way home (I already have the line, but don't use it). I tell her that if it happens again she should call 911 first, and then call me. She says she had wanted to but that she couldn't remember the apartment address in her panic and that's why she called me instead. We talk about how staying calm is really, really important. Then I print out a sheet with the apartment address and other important information on it and pin it to the wall. I leave to go to work, feeling comfortable that we have smoothed out the shortcomings that the emergency has highlighted.

I go downtown to my office and try to repair the cracks that have arisen from my absence of the past week. I don't get far. Around 2pm I get another frantic call from Norma.

'Calm down and tell me what's happening,' I plead.

'I think it's happening again,' she says, a little calmer, but still emotional. 'He didn't turn blue but he went very pale.'

'How is he now?' I ask.

'I think he's okay now.'

'Okay, I'll come right home,' I say, and hang up.

When I get to the apartment, Norma is in the lobby holding Evan. He looks like he is getting cold, but is otherwise his usual bright smiley self.

'Did you call an ambulance?' I ask, confused.

'No,' she says, 'but the apartment was too hot so we came out for air.'

We go upstairs and I show her how to turn the ceiling fan on.

We have another discussion about staying calm. Later, I take Evan out in the baby carrier and we buy a new phone, which I install when we get home.

Wednesday is fine. On Thursday morning, Norma calls me at work again, very calm this time.

'I think Evan is having a seizure,' she says. 'He keeps going into a kind of trance and making a tight fist. I took a video. He's okay right now.'

I hang up, make an appointment with the paediatrician for 2pm, and then call Norma back and tell her to bring Evan and meet me at the doctor's office.

The doctor listens to Norma describe everything she had seen, and then looks at the video.

'That's not a seizure,' he says, rubbing his greying beard, then fixing his yarmulke.

'A seizure has to have rhythmic movement of one or more limbs. That's missing here.'

Then he pulls out a large manual-like book, looks up the index, then turns to a page near the back of it.

'Breath-holding,' he says, 'Is a medical diagnosis.'

He spends the next twenty minutes or so reading aloud the pages of text the manual devotes to it. At various times Norma and I both chime in, saying things like, 'Ah, that makes sense' and 'Yes, that's exactly what happened.'

Then the doctor concludes, by the end of all this, that Evan must be working himself up to such a tizzy that he ends up holding his breath, causing him to turn blue. No lasting harm, just alarming, that's all.

Evan, Norma and I leave the doctor's surgery and cheerily walk the fifteen blocks back home. I feel buoyed by the diagnosis, almost ecstatic. It is a huge relief to be told that the only thing wrong with Evan is that he has a temper, and that the only thing to do is to sit and observe him during these breath-holding spells and, so long as it doesn't last more than a minute or so, let him ride it out.

As Norma and I chat en route I tell her she has done a great job of being observant, taking the video, and staying calm when she called me.

'Yes, but I used my mobile again!' she says.

We both laugh, and she promises to make use of the new land phone if she needs to call me again.

The next few weeks are just great. I feel so relieved that Evan's issues have turned out to be simple, and, after that very difficult and worrisome week, it is good to get back to enjoying him again.

A few weeks later, on a whim, I take Evan up to Woodstock in the Catskills region. A friend is going anyway, and nice weather is expected, so Evan and I catch a ride with her. When we get there, we all go to see another friend of ours, Stephanie, who sits in a little room at the back of the bookstore on the main street in town and reads tarot cards. Stephanie is a child of Woodstock Festival, although nowadays she has long white hair, which is balanced well by her red cowboy boots. My friend and I have both been getting tarot readings from Stephanie every year or so for many years now.

The great thing about Stephanie is that she is a very frugal psychic. In all the times I have had a reading from her, she has never told me one particular thing about the future. Instead, she gives general, and sometimes specific advice about how to navigate life over the next few months. ('Stop lingering on the past so much.' 'Join a group.' 'You don't really want a relationship so stop pretending that you do.' That kind of thing.) She says that if you are told what will happen, you will sit back and wait for it, rather than take the steps you are supposed to, to get there. 'The future can change,' she says.

She is delighted to see me walk in with Evan in my arms. I suppose I haven't been to see her since before I was pregnant. She sits with him on her knee for a long time and is clearly taken with him. Then she reads my cards.

I asked her generally if I am on the right track with Evan. She turns over one card, and speaks in reassuring tones, but then tells me to stop listening to the advice of others. Sometimes you can tell she is saying something that some higher force is telling her to say, and other times she is clearly just giving her own opinion. This was the former.

'What do you mean?' I ask.

She thinks for a moment, as if wondering what exactly these words mean.

'Take him into the bed with you when you sleep – he doesn't need to sleep on his own and neither do you. He's a good size now, just make sure he's safe.'

Then she adds, 'Your intuition is strong, so don't be swayed by what other people tell you. That includes me.'

We both laugh at this. She turns over another card.

'You are strong, which is good, because you are going to have to be so strong for Evan.'

This comes from a higher plane, too.

'Why?'

Again, she processes this, and speaking from her own opinion says, 'Well, he's going to be crawling soon, running around. It gets tough.'

Then she turns over the third card.

'Ah,' she says, more serious than before. 'This is very important. Do not listen to the devils that you meet. You will hear people insisting that you handle Evan their way, not yours. Listen to your own instinct. It's correct. Do not listen to the devils.'

I always treat these readings as a bit of harmless fun, interlaced with good advice that has worked well for me in the past. And I'm always pleased to see Stephanie. A few days after the Woodstock trip I read my horoscope for February. 'Get yourself a good lawyer,' it says. I post this on Facebook and it gets a good laugh from friends, as I am a lawyer.

I had always planned to get a babysitter for Evan. I have to work; there is no question of that. I have friends with children who send them to daycare centres or who have a selection of different babysitters because they don't want their child to become too attached to another adult. I have no qualms about that at all, though.

I am the youngest of five children, and by the time I came along, the others were already at school and my mum needed to go back to work. So my parents found a babysitter to come to our home and look after me. Her name was Connie Connolly and she was probably already close to retirement when we met, but she stayed with us for twelve years or so until old age got the better of her.

She was a lovely lady. She loved me deeply and I loved her. She used to warm my socks at the fire, before putting them on my feet. She would see me off to school in the morning and then still be there when I came home in the afternoon. I used to love following her around the house as she worked. She did all sorts of old-fashioned things like cleaning the brass work on the front door, polishing my dad's shoes each morning, and buffing up the silver tea set before everyone arrived home. We had a wonderful bond, but, as attached as I was to her, I always loved my parents more.

I was very proud of my parents. My dad was a doctor. He healed people, which was amazing. He was a general practitioner in the east end of Glasgow, at a time when it was a very rough and sometimes dangerous area. He loved it though. He used to take me to the Barras, which was a marketplace close to his surgery. It had a distinctive smell, the moister side of musty. Many of his patients had stalls there. They all greeted him like a demi-god, although he never indulged them in that.

Each time we went he would give me a fiver to spend. Then he would make me spend at least half of it on buying something for my mum and for Connie from some of the people he knew. I cherish those memories of us hanging out together at the Barras. Ironically, for a doctor, he himself became ill when I was still young. By the time I was in my teens he had retired and become a recluse. He basically lost interest in everything, including, it felt, me. It was part of his illness, but it was beyond my comprehension at the time.

I remained very close to my mum. I'm sure dad's illness was very hard on her but she was always cheerful and very, very loving. She was a high-school teacher. She taught English. Occasionally, when it was appropriate, she would let me come to school with her. I saw how wonderful she was at her job. Everybody liked her. More than that, I saw her in her element. She was great at teaching and she knew it. It was easy to keep her on a pedestal. She inspired me. She made me work hard by making me realise that I enjoyed working hard. She encouraged me to do whatever I wanted with my life, though, so long as it was really what I wanted.

I went to university in Glasgow and had a blast there. At the end – the very end – I worked hard and got a decent degree. Then I worked in a restaurant for a couple of years, because it was great fun. Then, on a trip to the States to see my brother and oldest sister (both of whom had moved there a few years before) I fell in love with San Francisco. There was no going back. Well, I did go back, but only to quit my job, break up with my boyfriend, and wait for a visa to come through. At the age of

Our Beginnings

twenty-four I moved to San Francisco with $700 in my pocket and a heart full of hope.

I spent five happy years there. I got in with a wonderful group of friends, mostly Irish. Those were the dot-com years, and San Francisco was at the heart of the prosperity boom. Anyone and everyone could make a fortune if they wanted, things were so good. None of us cared about any of that, though. We all worked jobs that didn't inspire us, and didn't pay much, but allowed us enough free time to get the most out of life. We went biking, went on camping trips, hiked and, most of all, socialised. I think we all recognised that we had a very special friendship, in a very special time and place. Eventually, as we all began to nudge thirty, most of us moved on. Some went travelling around the world, some home to Ireland.

I decided to go to Washington, DC and attend law school. Violet, a great friend and room-mate, opted to move to New York at the same time. The two of us drove across country together to start our new lives apart. As we have boasted ever since, we did so without a map, and in the days before sat navs. All we had was a guidebook that recommended certain routes (no freeways, just two-lane highways at the most) and offered topologically drawn maps. Violet became adept at measuring distances by taking a piece of string and marking the drawings with it, then measuring the length of the string against the scale given on the page and making the necessary calculations. She got it right every time and earned the moniker 'Violet the Co-Pilot'. At the end of the trip we said goodbye at JFK airport. She went to live in Queens, New York, and I went to live in Adams Morgan, Washington, DC.

Law was something I had always wanted to do. I suppose I started my law degree later in life because I needed the years in between to grow up a bit. To say the transition between fun-filled hippy-reminiscing San Francisco and buttoned-down Washington, DC – especially law school there – was tough is an understatement.

I really didn't enjoy my time in DC. American law schools are notoriously difficult. The coursework was intense, and usually bewildering, at least at first. I possibly had it a little harder than other students because I hadn't grown up learning about the American Constitution and other American values. Eventually, though, I got the hang of it.

After graduation I passed the New York bar exam and moved to New York City. I arrived there eleven months after the attacks of 9/11, in 2001. The city was still in shock, and also in recession after the burst of the dot-com bubble. It was hard to get a job, particularly as I refused to apply to any of the big law firms. There was no point. Even if I got hired, I'm not a very good team player (which you have to be in those places) and I'm not very good at being told what to do (another 'must'). Anyway, I wanted court experience, and you don't get within earshot of a courtroom for many years if you work for a big firm.

I took a job in a small 'boutique' law firm, as my boss called it. Actually he would take any and every case of any type so long as it paid, so I think 'boutique' is stretching it a bit. That initial misrepresentation of his should have been a warning for me. He eventually went to jail for defrauding his clients. A colleague, Neil Schreffler, had been a sole practitioner before coming to work at our firm and when the boss's indiscretions became known Neil jumped ship and took me with him. Together, and with absolutely no capital (as the move had been so sudden), we started the law firm of Schreffler Schwarz.

We may have had no money (and no clients at first) but we had a wonderful relationship together. Neil made me laugh every single day. But, crucially, he could switch into serious mode and give me all the advice I asked him for, professionally and perfectly. Neil taught me absolutely everything I needed to know about running a practice, getting clients, and about how to practice law as best as possible. Eventually we realised that our areas of interest in the law were too diverse to enjoy the economies of scale that a partnership is meant to bring. Very amicably, we split, him to a law firm, and me to my own sole practice, though he remained my good friend and mentor.

Starting a solo practice was difficult; I can't deny it. It took me a year and a half to get into profit (and stop sinking further into debt). It took me a little longer than that to not be absolutely terrified of my job. Eventually, though, things worked out. As I grew in caseload and successes, I also grew in confidence. I joined a networking group (BNI Chapter 12) in Manhattan, which enabled me to make connections I didn't have before (because I didn't grow up or attend school in New York). I practised mostly in commercial litigation and, because people expected it of me as a foreign lawyer, some immigration.

In my first year as a lawyer (at the 'boutique' firm) I took on many *pro bono* cases. It wasn't entirely altruistic. I knew that it was the fastest route to getting as much court experience as possible (I was a courtroom addict and there wasn't enough to satisfy me in the paid cases at the firm). My very first *pro bono* case was an asylum application from a lesbian from Saudi Arabia. I threw myself into that case and became good friends with the client. In the midst of it, I realised I was being a hypocrite: I was gay too and I was pretending I wasn't. I had come out in San Francisco years before, but our group of friends (who were mostly straight) was more about friendship, and none of us really sought romance. When I went to law school, for reasons I still haven't ever really worked out, I decided I 'wanted to be straight', and went back into the closet. Even writing that now, sixteen or so years later, my head is starting to ache at remembering the horrendous battle that raged within me every single day, trying to be something God had never intended me to be. So, at the age of thirty-one, I came out of the closet, again. After we had won the asylum case and the client was allowed to remain in the USA (and not go back to Saudi Arabia, where she would be crushed to death for her sexuality), we went for a drink. She wanted to pay as a 'thank you'. We ended up splitting the bill since we both had reasons to thank each other.

I tried a few relationships, got my heart broken a few times, and then I tried therapy. There, I discovered many things about myself, two of which are relevant here:

1. I wanted to be a mother
2. I wanted to be a single mother

It's not that I had a huge urge to do it alone but seeing how relationships can collapse no matter how hard you work at them, I had no real belief that having a partner would work out. Sharing a child with someone who lived somewhere else was something I could not bear to think about. I already knew that I would love my children so much that the threat of not having them full-time, in my home with me, was too much to bear.

After sixteen months of fertility treatment and many vials of donor sperm, I eventually conceived. Evan Louis Schwarz was born on 3 September 2011 in Manhattan. It was, and still is, the happiest day of my life.

We bonded immediately. I've heard of other parents taking some time, but I loved my son immensely from the moment he was placed in my arms.

Our first couple of days alone in the apartment were quite nervy for me, but in less than a week Evan and I were a wonderful team. He was a very placid baby. I'd known from carrying him that he would be. He never kicked hard and he moved very gently as he grew inside me.

He was an early smiler – he had the most beautiful broad grin. After a short time, he began to chuckle. It didn't have to be at something funny, I think he just liked the feeling of it. Me too. He slept well and ate well.

Because Evan was such a good baby, I had a relatively easy time of it. I really didn't ever want for sleep. My milk was good and flowed well for him. And I was so madly deeply in love with him. The rushes of love caught me by surprise. Sometimes I would wonder how it could be that I could possibly love him even more than I did the day before. I was intensely happy.

In Evan's first few weeks I took him down to my office a few times if I had to do something there that I couldn't do at home. He mostly slept as I worked, but I hoped eventually, in the years to come, to achieve with him what my mum had achieved with me. I wanted him to know his mum worked very hard and tried to help people. Most of all, I wanted him to know that all of my efforts, ultimately, were for him.

As soon as Evan's passport came through I took him back to Glasgow for a visit. I had allowed myself two months of maternity leave (although I still did plenty of work from home while Evan slept). I wanted him to meet his grandparents, and I could work as easily from Glasgow as I could from my apartment.

Mum was delighted to meet her ninth grandchild. She held him for hours. I had to ask for him back more than once. My dad wasn't at home when we arrived. He had been quite ill for some time and was in hospital. He had never emerged from his reclusiveness in the twenty-six years since he retired, although we had all adjusted to it. In the first two weeks that Evan and I were in Glasgow, though, he was incredibly sociable and alert each time I visited him. He was confined to his hospital bed, but he looked and sounded very bright. For those two weeks, he was the dad that I had lost all those years ago. And then he died. At least he met Evan.

The day before Dad's funeral I took Evan shopping for something to wear. We were in Gap looking around and a song started playing on the store's speakers. 'This is a song sent from your granddad to me,' I told Evan. I was sure of it, even though I didn't recognise the song from the first few bars. Gradually as it went on, I realised it was Willie Nelson, singing, 'Always On My Mind'. 'Maybe I didn't hold you, all those lonely lonely times, and I guess I never told you, I'm so happy that you're mine.' This and the other verses resonated so completely with me as a message from my dad. I was very grateful for it.

After the funeral, Evan and I stayed an extra two weeks to settle my mum into her new routine alone at home. She herself was very frail by this point, although she was mentally sharp as a tack, as she had always been. Several years ago, she had an illness that seemed to add twenty years to her overnight. We arranged for her to have a series of carers to come in several times a day to give her meals and do her shopping for her. This was by now a well-established routine for her. It didn't feel very good to have to leave her, but Evan and I couldn't put off going back to New York any longer. Work was piling up and I had a series of court appearances to attend. And I still hadn't organised day care for Evan.

When I was pregnant, my obstetrician introduced me to her own babysitter, Clare. The family were moving upstate and Clare needed to find a new position. We met and Clare was every bit as nice as my doctor had promised. She babysat Evan a couple of times in the first month, and fell completely in love with him. It was a great match. The only problem was that she could only work three days a week. She was an artist, and very dedicated to not letting that side of her life slide. We decided she would babysit for the occasional night out, but that I would get someone else for the four days a week that I really needed.

Just before I left Scotland, I got an email from Jackie Frank, a close friend, and also president of my networking group. She had a lead about a nanny looking for a family. Her name was Norma Leonce. Jackie sent me a fairly long letter of recommendation from her current family. Jodi, the mother, had written that she was very fond of Norma and so was her one-year-old son, Jeremy, but that she had decided to become a stay-at-home mum and therefore didn't need Norma any more. To soften the blow, she was trying to set her up with a new family.

I emailed Jodi directly and got more information from her about Norma, all of which sounded good. She gave me Norma's number and I gave her a call. I explained who I was, how I had her number, and we set up a meeting for the day after Evan and I returned to New York.

So, in early November, Norma knocked on our door and entered our lives. She was young (twenty-six), dark-skinned, a little taller than me and a little stout. She explained she was originally from St Lucia, in the Caribbean, and had been in New York for about eight years. She had looked after newborns and infants her entire adult life. The interview went well. Norma held Evan throughout and he seemed very comfortable in her arms. She had a warm and easy laugh.

Based on this meeting and Jodi's extensive and glowing reference, as well as our emails, I hired Norma and we wrote out a schedule to take us through to the Christmas holidays. I explained that Evan and I would be going back to Scotland for three weeks over Christmas and New Year and she said she was fine with that. She said that she could easily pick up babysitting hours from other families that she did occasional work for.

Evan and I went home to Scotland for Christmas, where we had a week of extended family (my three sisters, Anne, Frances and Pauline, and their offspring) all staying together in the family home with Mum. We had several nice outings, including the Scottish Christmas staples of carnival and pantomime. We also scattered Dad's ashes around the garden on Christmas Eve, a beautiful sunny wintry day, with the smell of wood-burning fires in the air. Dad had lived in that house for forty-five years, and it felt very fitting.

As usual it was the new generation – my nephews Angus, seventeen, Finlay, fourteen, and my nieces Eleonor, ten, and Lucia, seven – who stole the show with their liveliness and cheeriness. This year was, of course, very special, because Evan too became a part of the entertainment. He seemed to take his first Christmas in his stride.

The day after Christmas there was a huge windy, blustery storm. That evening Evan and I were getting ready to go to a party. We kept getting delayed. He needed a feed. Then he needed changing. Then his clothes got soiled and I had to change them too. Eventually we were ready. Just as we were leaving the house the big old silver birch tree in the front garden came crashing down, right across the driveway. It was a hundred years old, massive and weighed a ton. And it missed us by seconds.

It took ten men most of the night to cut away at it and move the pieces off the path. We were all quite shocked and even upset at losing it, but no one was injured and that was the most important thing.

We ended up staying at home that evening. We literally could not get out of the driveway because of the tree. The following week, though, we went out to a New Year party. As we stood in the cold evening air, both wrapped up, me holding Evan close in the baby carrier, I marvelled at how lucky I was to have someone so delicious to kiss at midnight.

A few days later we took a short trip to Madrid to see Pauline and her family. Although we had just seen each other it was lovely to see them again in their own home. Evan brought as many smiles to Spanish faces as he had done in Glasgow and New York. My 'wean in Spain', as I kept calling him, never failed to make me proud.

NEW YEAR, NEW YORK

We got back to New York, and on 10 January 2012, Norma came to work four days a week on a permanent basis. I hoped to go home to Scotland for a long weekend every six weeks, as I had been doing since my parents aged. Norma and I agreed that she would be paid for the week we were away, but would give me an extra day of work the week before and the week after. It was a good deal for both of us.

It didn't take long for us to work out a pretty good routine. She would arrive at 8am and I would leave and go downtown to my office. I would text her several times a day and she would let me know how things were going. Around 5.30pm I would head back up town to the apartment. While it was difficult to be away from Evan (more so than I had anticipated), I always loved coming home to him. Sometimes just thinking about him, I'd burst with pride and happiness. I used to wish I'd run into people I hadn't seen in a few years so I could tell them all I couldn't stop and talk, I had to run home to my wonderful baby – the best baby in the world. Norma was supposed to leave at 6pm every day, but most days she would stay a little longer, just to chat about Evan for a while. That was just fine by me: Evan was so much more important to me than anything else in the world that all I wanted to talk about was him. He was certainly pretty much all I could think about anyway, both at home and at work.

Norma was very knowledgeable about babies. As well as her eight years of experience, she had gone on a baby-nursing course a year or two before. Her experience was hugely beneficial for me because I could ask her questions and she had answers. Sometimes she would come in the next day with more information because she had gone home and done some research on it. She told me she wanted to be a paediatrician.

After the 'ALTE' incident, and in the weeks that followed, I grew more and more at ease with Norma. She had good boundaries, which I liked, and she was never overly inquisitive of my private life. She was really good with Evan, and she continued to be a good source of information for me, when I needed it. I started to consider myself as lucky to find her as my own family had been with Connie Connolly.

Part Two

Everything Changes

Things settled down again and everything seemed to be going well. I took on a couple of new cases and my law practice was back up at the level it had been before my maternity leave. Evan continued to grow, bigger and more beautiful, every day. He learned to roll over and could almost sit on his own. He started to eat solids, and suddenly an excess of peas and carrots filled our mealtimes together.

One Thursday afternoon in mid-February, I came home early from work, let Norma leave, and then enjoyed a lovely evening with Evan. We went out for our nightly walk up and down the streets of the Upper West Side, enjoying strangers' pleasantries. I don't recall having random conversations with strangers before I had a baby, but with Evan strapped to my chest in the baby carrier I can hardly walk a Manhattan block without someone stopping to chat.

That night, when we get back home to our little studio apartment, there is a brown paper package tied up in string – literally – waiting for us. A friend's mother has sent Evan a Scottish dolly, specially knitted for him. It is a lovely gift to get, with its rosy cheeks painted with lipstick, and its body tightly stuffed with stockings. I sit it next to Evan, who by now is in his yellow ducky night suit. I take lots of photographs, all of them with Evan smiling dutifully and beautifully. Then Evan and I hang out on the couch until it is time for bed. I have stopped trying to impose a bedtime on him and have also taken Stephanie's advice and now sleep with him in bed beside me. The result is a lot less tears, and a cosy and pleasant sleep for us both.

The next morning I wake up to Evan smiling at me. They are the biggest smiles I've ever seen. He is beyond adorable; I could eat him up. Norma arrives around 8am and I reluctantly say goodbye to Evan again. He isn't even crying when I leave – just smiling the sweetest smile. It will haunt me every day since that I didn't ditch work that day and stay at home with him.

I can't, though – I have an arbitration hearing in an office in Times Square and there is no getting out of it. Throughout the day I send a few sneaky texts to Norma asking how things are – everything is apparently fine. The hearing ends early, around 2.30pm. It is a beautiful day, especially for February in New York. It has been a mild winter, but even so, this is exceptionally sunny and even almost balmy – about as good as it gets for this time of year. I really feel like going home and taking Evan to the park, but then I think about how tight money is and how I could fit in a couple of billable hours if I go back to the office. Besides, I went home early yesterday. So I go downtown to my office instead of uptown to our studio apartment.

I stay at the office for a couple of hours, and when I finally leave I run a couple of errands and then take the subway to our stop on 72nd Street. Before going home, though, I go in to the camera shop nearby to print out the gorgeous photos of Evan with the Scottish doll. As I wait for the machine to deliver the prints, I look at my phone.

There is a text from Norma.

'Can you please call me, Evan is holding his breath for a really long time.'

I run.

It seems to take an age to get the block and a half to our building. I run into the elevator and it goes directly to our floor. I run down the hallway to our apartment, and hammer on the door as I fumble for my keys. When I get inside, I see Evan's stroller. No one is home. The living area is in a state of disarray.

I run out of the apartment, back downstairs, and am running through the lobby when Norma calls my phone again.

'Is he breathing?' I scream.

'It's really bad. They can't get a pulse,' she cries.

I am already out on the street by this point, frantically running without knowing where to. Then a lady comes on the phone. She is much calmer. She says, 'Your son is very sick, and you need to come straight here to St Luke's. He is very, very sick.'

I jump in a cab and get there in about five minutes. I run to the front desk and shout into the air, 'Where's my baby?'

'Take her to RESUS.'

I am taken to a doorway of a large room. A half dozen paramedics stand in a row, staring at something I can't see. A big fair-haired fireman comes over to me and holds me firmly by my upper arms and says, 'We received a call to your apartment. When we got there your son wasn't breathing and we couldn't get a pulse. We tried to resuscitate him and we brought him here. They're working on him now. You can't go in yet.'

I hear myself scream, 'Let me see my baby!'

A lady comes and puts her arm around me – probably the lady I spoke to on the phone. She leads me into a room, where Norma is sitting, crying.

'What happened?'

'He stopped breathing,' she says through sobs.

'We'd been at home all day and I went to get his bottle and I heard a scream and he stopped breathing.'

Then the lady comes back and tells me I can see Evan now. She walks me back to the same room and the FDNY guys are just leaving, and looking more relaxed than when I'd seen them a few minutes before.

I see Evan. He is lying on the table, with a tube down his throat, and a hospital gown on. He is breathing strangely, big breaths, about three seconds apart.

They tell me I can touch him, but not to pick him up. I hug him as he lies there.

He is entirely motionless.

'Evan! Come on, Evan! Evan!' I start shouting.

The lady says, 'Yes, that's it, try and see if you can wake him.'

I can't, though.

After a few minutes of standing over him, I am asked to wait outside while they prepare him for tests. Norma is already there; she has been joined by her sister.

'It was on my watch,' she keeps saying, nearly hysterical.

I say, 'Norma, I trust you so much, it's not your fault.'

They send Evan for a CT scan. As we wait, Norma and her sister sit holding each other on the bench across from mine.

They bring him back, wheeling him past us, and into a bay in the main part of the ER. Another doctor has started her shift and is attending to him. 'I want to put a central line in,' I can hear her say.

Another doctor, a tall Asian man with glasses, calls me over to where he is standing, at the reception desk.

'We got the CT scan results back and you and I need to talk with the other doctor, and when we do, it needs to be out of the presence of the babysitter.'

'What's wrong with Evan?' I ask him, with urgency in my voice. It seems so cruel to make me wait.

The female doctor is busy inserting a long catheter into the skin at the top of Evan's right thigh. Once she is done, the Asian doctor takes me over to her. Norma is standing about ten feet away, still being held by her sister. The Asian doctor looks over at her, and then turns to me and quietly says, 'The CT scan is abnormal. It's Shaken Baby Syndrome. It's the babysitter, she was with him.'

I have no idea what to do or say or even think. I have heard of Shaken Baby Syndrome – they make every new parent watch a video about it before they are allowed to take their baby home from hospital – but I don't know what it means for Evan. I look at my baby boy, lying on the table, with so many tubes coming out of his body. I can't speak; I can't cry.

'The police will get involved, and it's very important that you don't interfere with their investigation. Do you understand?' says the female doctor.

I don't recall responding.

'Don't tip the babysitter off. Don't tell her anything about a diagnosis. You can't get in the way of what the police need to do,' one of them continues.

They tell me they are transferring Evan to the Intensive Care Unit at Columbia University NY Presbyterian Hospital. Norma comes over to me after the doctors have turned back to Evan and she asks me what is happening. I tell her they are moving him to another hospital, but that they don't know yet what is wrong.

'I'll come with you,' she says.

I really do not want her to.

A little while later, a new group of paramedics arrive and prepare Evan for transport. A new doctor has arrived to accompany us on the journey.

'I know this is overwhelming for you,' she offers, 'but we will take good care of him.'

I don't know it is overwhelming, I just know I feel numb and I have no idea what to do.

Norma comes over with her bag. The paramedic and the

female doctor speak at the same time, both telling her that there is only room for one adult in the ambulance.

'Just go home. I'll call you when I know something,' I tell her.

She accepts this. Then she pulls my house keys and Evan's pacifier from her pocket and hands them both to me. 'I'll see you on Tuesday,' she says, as though everything will be back to normal by then.

I sit in the front passenger seat of the ambulance as the doctor and a paramedic sit with Evan in the back. We drive up the West Side Highway in silence. I really don't have a thought in my head. Every now and then I can hear a siren and I look around for an ambulance. Then I remember: we are travelling in it.

The ambulance takes us to the ICU at Columbia University NY Presbyterian Hospital on 168th Street. We are wheeled into a room just one floor below where Evan was born, five and a half months ago. His birth was the best experience of my life and I have always associated Columbia University NY Presbyterian Hospital with the happiest of thoughts.

We are taken to the ICU on the ninth floor. A nurse tells me to wait outside as they see to Evan, and leads me to a waiting area by the elevators. There is a computer nearby, for public use. I sit down and start searching for clues about Shaken Baby Syndrome (SBS). I don't like what I find: swelling of the brain, bleeding of the brain, retinal damage. Then, brain damage, cerebral palsy, often death. A third die, a third have serious brain damage, and a third don't have any lasting damage. God, let it be the third option, please, please, please.

I email a friend, Deborah, who lives nearby. She comes over

and sits with me for the interminable time I have to wait. In retrospect these hours of not knowing, and of not being able to process anything, are the easy part.

While we sit waiting, two men approach me and introduce themselves as officers of Child Protective Services, or ACS (Administration for Children's Services) as it's known in New York. They ask me to follow them into a small relatives' room, known as the 'green room', just past the elevators.

I do, and the three of us sit down. They ask many questions about me, about Evan, and about what has happened to get us to where we are now. I tell them as much as I can. I show them the texts Norma and I exchanged that day, where she told me that Evan was laughing with her, that he was eating normally. Later, I can't recall all that much about what was said, but I remember trying to be as helpful as possible.

Eventually, I am allowed back in to see Evan. He is trussed up, with tubes and sensors everywhere. He looks tiny and very pale. The doctor, a blonde woman with dancing eyes, says to me, 'I have to tell you, I can't guarantee he will survive. The first seventy-two hours are crucial and he might not get through them.'

I feel my eyes widen, but I can't speak.

Another doctor comes in, a youngish guy in a lab coat. He explains to the female doctor, and to me (as though I am just another member of staff), that the CT scan shows old and new blood, indicating days and days of shaking. His tone is nonchalant and casual, and his hands remain in his pockets the entire time. I can't believe what I am hearing.

Everything Changes

The doctors step out and I stand there, now alone, with Evan. I am in my stockinged feet and my suit from the day at work. I keep thinking about how the next few days could take him.

My brother Anton happens to call me from California. I break the news to him and tell him what I can. I can hear the shock in his breath and his wife in the background asking, 'Is he dead?'

I can't cope with the call after that and hand the phone to Deborah, who has come in to see Evan. She explains what she can to him. When she gets off the phone she tells me that Anton is on his way on the next available flight.

I call Pauline, in Madrid. By this time it is probably 7am over there. She answers the phone, 'Yes?', in a frantic tone. Perhaps she can still recall the phone call just a few months earlier from another sister, to tell her that our dad was dying.

'It's Evan. He's very, very sick. He might not make it.'

Then I call my sister Anne in England, who is, coincidentally, driving up to see Mum in Glasgow. Then I call Mum. I'm really not sure what any of them say to me in response, but they all know that it is touch and go with Evan.

Deborah leaves at some point well into the night, promising to come back in a few hours. Eventually, and at the urging of the nurses on duty, I lie down to sleep on the little cot bed next to Evan's, holding his blue dinosaur-covered snowsuit close to me, smelling his scent. Mostly I toss and turn and every now and then a voice in my head says, 'He's going to die'. All I can do is internally scream at myself. Scream and scream, 'Don't you dare lose faith in him, don't you dare give up!' But those thoughts sneak in again and again. I remember the flight we have booked to Scotland for the following Friday, and wonder if I will be on it with a little white coffin. I spend hours swiping this and other bad thoughts away.

I focus on the bigger tree that had fallen down in my mum's front garden a few months ago. I try to keep thinking that if God wanted to take Evan this would have been his opportunity. Surely he wouldn't have spared either of us then, only to come back for Evan seven weeks later? But then I remember the second tree that came down, just a month ago, when Evan was in hospital. I try not to draw any hysterical conclusions, and put thoughts of 'omens' out of my mind as much as I can. I say a prayer, among all my praying for Evan, that I won't get word of the third and final tree in that garden coming down. Just in case.

Dawn breaks to reveal a view of the Hudson River and New Jersey. I walk over to the parents' area on the east side, pour a cup of bad coffee from a machine, and stand at the windows. The view on this side is the same view I had looked out on when I was in labour, five and a half months before.

The doctor with the sparkly eyes comes back in to Evan's room just as I return. I buttonhole her. 'What are his chances? Tell me something positive – you can't just tell me negative things – there has to be something to hope for.'

'Okay,' she says, 'he has a reasonable chance of survival. I have seen kids this sick recover but I don't think I've ever seen a kid this non-responsive.'

She asks me for more information. I tell her about the first hospitalisation, about the later visits to the doctor. I tell her about Evan's paediatrician and that he had said the video of Evan taken by Norma didn't show Evan having a seizure because there was no rhythmic movement.

'That's not correct,' she tells me. 'You can seize without any movement at all.'

I tell her how Evan cries often when I leave in the mornings. 'I think he's too young to cry because of separation anxiety. He may have been crying because he was scared of your babysitter,' she tells me.

Then she walks out of the room and the gravity of her final sentence leaves me staring into space.

A new doctor arrives to take over for the day shift. She has long silver hair and wears a lilac sweater. The first thing she says to me is, 'Your son has a very serious injury, and it can only have been another person that did this to him. I'm not making any judgements here, but this is what it is.'

I sit there, frozen. 'Just bring him back to me,' I reply.

Various doctors come by to ask me more questions. They introduce themselves by speciality: Heart. Haematology. Surgery.

Later, a police officer, Detective Reyes, shows up. Short, with long hair, she is wearing plain clothes and a dark trench coat. She asks me more detailed questions than the ACS officers have, and certainly seems to be more attuned to the situation. At one point I start to get very upset about Norma, and how this could have been going on without my knowing it.

'Why did I leave him with her?' I say, through heavy tears.

'You didn't do anything that any other caring mother wouldn't have done. This is not your fault,' she says.

When she is finished with the interview she says, 'I want you to know that, if I can, I will do everything possible to bring this woman to justice.'

I go back in to Evan, who hasn't changed any: he is still unconscious. I am still not allowed to hold him.

By this time I have already texted a few friends to tell them what is going on. My friend Liz shows up very early. She lives in Brooklyn, so she must have come as soon as she heard. Deborah comes back, and the three of us sit out on the chairs in the lobby.

Two doctors come by on their way to the elevators. They see me and stop to talk, introducing themselves as 'The Neurologists'. I stand to talk with them, still in my stockinged feet and by now very crumpled suit. The male, younger of the two, Indian and with a satchel slung across his chest, doesn't say anything. The female doctor is a portly lady with beady eyes. She has a white coat on and her purse is draped over her shoulder. They both look like they are on their way to lunch. She goes into a long explanation of everything they have found wrong with Evan. After some time she says, with more animation than before, 'But none of that is the issue – the real issue, which we haven't paid enough attention to, is the bleeding in his brain. My guess is that will continue to develop.'

I am taken aback by her change of tone, from informative to almost excited. It doesn't seem to gel with the news she is telling me, that she thinks Evan is going to get worse.

'But is it possible it has stopped?' I manage to ask.

She says, 'It's possible, but it's more likely to be compounded, so by this time tomorrow I feel it will be confirmed and his brain will die. Then we will discuss switching off the machines.'

She gives me a small nod of something short of sympathy, and then turns on her heel and goes off to lunch.

I sit down, feeling every ounce of energy leave my body. There is not a thought in my head. I feel a shroud of darkness, an emptiness, overcome me.

Deborah and Liz sit either side of me. 'I can't lose him,' I remember saying, eventually. I know they both say consoling things to me but I don't remember any of it.

I somehow find the wherewithal to call all the family again, and tell them what the neurologist has told me. 'I'm sorry,' is all I can hear them say. All I can feel is anger that none of them can change this.

I go back in to sit with Evan, wondering if these moments will be our last together. It is too much to bear. I call Pauline again.

'I can't do this.'

'Yes you can,' she says, 'You have to be strong for Evan.'

She is right: Evan needs me. I pull myself together as much as I can.

An hour or so later, a different doctor walks in, reading Evan's file.

'We will send him for an MRI [Magnetic Resonance Imaging] scan on Tuesday or Wednesday when he's more stable – that will give us more of an idea about what is going on,' he tells me, not looking up from his notes.

Another gear change; I can hardly keep up. I stare at the doctor. Finally he looks up at me.

'But it doesn't look like we are going to get to Tuesday, does it?' I say.

He looks puzzled, so I tell him about the conversation with The Neurologists at the elevator.

'I apologise if any doctor here gave you a conclusion at this early stage in our investigations. I'm not saying that what she explained will definitely not happen, but we absolutely can't conclude that right now.'

Suddenly hope steps right back into our lives. It feels so much better than the despair that had taken its place for the last couple of hours.

After this, I stop every single person who comes in to look at or treat Evan and say to them, 'The only way this is going to end is with my boy coming back to me. If you don't believe in his full recovery then you are not to touch him.'

I make each of them promise me that yes, they are 100 per cent devoted to his full recovery. One or two tried to sneak in disclaimers, like 'to the extent that is possible', but all of them promise.

My brother Anton arrives from California in the afternoon. Deborah comes back with Jackie. I tell Jackie that the doctors suspect Norma has hurt Evan. I can see the blood drain from her face. Jackie had been the one to find the advertisement Norma's previous employer had posted. It is a tiny and tenuous link from there to here. Jackie is blameless. Besides, I interviewed Norma and checked her references, and I had also very much grown to trust her.

Later, in a steady flow, a whole bunch of people show up. Jackie has rallied together everyone we are friends with through the networking chapter we are part of, and friends from other avenues of life come too. Pretty soon, the waiting area by the elevators is filled with around twenty people. They bring clothes, coffee, cakes, toothpaste, deodorant, rosary beads and anything else they think might help.

I call my mum several more times that first full day. Sometimes the reception on my phone fails, and I can hear her, but she can't hear me. On these occasions she just says beautifully consoling, tender things into the receiver, hoping I can hear them, which I do. She would come to New York, she says, if it would do any good. But we both know that it's not possible: she is too old and frail to make the journey.

Jackie went to the camera shop where I had abandoned Evan's photographs the day before. They had been handed in and were behind the counter, so she paid for them and brought them to the hospital. Various friends set about taping them up all around Evan's room, so the nurses and doctors can see what they are working for.

Two more friends arrive, and when they see Evan they both start crying. 'No, you can't do that in here,' I tell them instinctively. It doesn't seem fair on Evan to have people in despair. The mood around him must be positive and loving, and not negative in any way.

Almost as soon as these friends have gone, I get a text from another friend offering me his 'heartfelt sympathy'. I have to text back asking only for positivity. I am not trying to be ungrateful, but I am still trying to muster strength, and there feels something very vulnerable in sympathy. I can't risk feeling sorry for myself if I want to keep strong for Evan.

I become aware that I have yet to cry. I am in shock and perhaps these kind friends are not. Perhaps it isn't fair to ask them not to show negative emotions. I can't afford to care.

During the night, around 2am, Evan's heart rate suddenly plummets. Five medics arrive within seconds. A crash cart is quickly rolled in. A red-haired doctor puts two small paddles on Evan's tiny bare chest and then shocks him twice. Evan's torso lifts up both times. Evan's heart rate is back to a safe rate.

It is over in three minutes. In that time I have said a decade of the rosary a friend brought for me. If ever there was a decade of a rosary put to good use it is in those three minutes. It distracted me and stopped me thinking any more of those horrendous negative thoughts from the night before.

Once it's over, the red-haired doctor (who introduces himself as Patrick) sits next to me and asks if I have any questions. He is young but serious and I can tell by the way he has just handled the situation that he is both experienced and invested in Evan's wellbeing.

'Just bring my boy back,' I tell him.

'We can't bring back the brain cells that have already been damaged,' he says gently.

'I know, but do what you can to help the ones he has left.'

'We'll do our very best for him,' he says, with sincerity.

I don't sleep much after that. Instead I fill up on more machine coffee and call Pauline again. Then I call Anne, who by now is with our mum in Glasgow. Liz and another friend arrive at the hospital early, around 9am. We sit at the tables in the parents' area. After a few minutes of talking, I suddenly break down. I sob and sob and sob. It is the first time I have cried.

PRAYING

I would say I am spiritual, but not religious. Organised religion has never really appealed to me. I have always had a very strong belief in God, though. And I have always prayed, but never according to any kind of structure. I've always felt prayer is an intensely personal thing. I couldn't even tell you which of my friends or relatives do it. But in this time, I know it is the only thing that anyone can do to help. So whenever anyone asks what they can do for us, I tell them to pray as hard as they can.

I pray with Evan too. This morning, when we are alone, I tell him that if he wants to go to heaven now, his granddad will take very good care of him until I get there too, but if he can, I would love for him to stay on earth with me.

Later, in the afternoon, a Catholic priest from Africa and a Buddhist monk, both from the hospital's pastoral care service, come to see us. They listen to what is going on and ask if they can say a prayer over Evan, which I appreciate.

The Catholic priest says I should get Evan christened immediately. I say no, that I will hold off with the hope that we will get through this and have the big party I had always planned for it. The priest doesn't think much of the idea, but I know it is important to keep that goal.

I ask them to pray for Norma too. I tell them, 'I don't know what happened, but I think she must be going through a terrible time right now. Even if she did this, whether it was deliberate or not, I would still like her to be prayed for.'

When Monday arrives, the hospital becomes busier as the working week starts. More students come in to see Evan, more touching and prodding and writing of notes. New nurses, new doctors. Still no movement from Evan.

Early in the morning I have a visit from two more ACS caseworkers. One, Ms Dominique, is a tall woman, with dyed blonde hair. The other one, a lady whose name I never learn, has very large, almost comical, magnified glasses. We sit in the green room and they ask me question after question. The bespectacled one becomes so confused and mixed up with the facts that we have to go over each point again and again. The interview only lasts half an hour or so. It seems unlikely they could have gathered much to work on, but they tell me they are done, and off they go.

I go back to Evan's room, but not for long. Almost immediately I have a visit from a short French woman with a curly bob. She introduces herself as Dr Jocelyn Brown, an investigative doctor from the Child Advocacy Center (CAC), which is attached to the hospital.

Dr Brown invites me back to the green room, where she and her assistant interview me at length. By now, Evan and I have been assigned a social worker, called Soulemar. She comes too, and so does Anton.

Everything Changes

It is an awful experience. I am tired and I am devastated and the last thing I want to do is talk about it. Nonetheless, Dr Brown needs to know. She is probing but gentle. I tell the entire story again but, thanks to her professionalism in asking the right questions, I am able to go into far greater detail than before. I feel the need to explain why I hadn't gone home early on Friday afternoon, but had gone back to my office instead. I explain that if I am not working, I am with Evan; I am happiest when I am with him. As I speak, I wonder why on earth had I felt the need to go back to work that day? How different things might have been if I had only chosen to walk uptown in the sunshine to my boy, instead of getting on a train and going downtown.

After an hour or so of giving as much information as possible, it gets too much. I ask everyone to leave and to turn the lights off. I sit there for hours, crying in the darkened room. Suddenly I want my dad. I want him here, healthy, strong, smart and with medical answers. But Dad is dead. Anyway, it had been decades since he showed any interest in talking about medicine, or anything else really. I want to go back, all the way back, thirty years if I must, to a time when everything still made sense. If dreams are allowed then I might as well dream big.

Friends come and go. There is an air of exultation when we make it past the seventy-two-hour waiting period, and the danger of further bleeding becomes less. I am aware, though, that this sets us on a new course. With more tests due in the next few days, we have to hope the damage to Evan's brain isn't too bad.

My prayer becomes, 'Dear God, please give us enough brain activity to work with.'

At some point in those first few days, a friend brings me a notebook and a couple of pens. 'It might help if you write things down,' she tells me…

21 February 2012

Evan is hooked up to a catheter that draws the urine from his bladder because his body has stopped being able to expel it. I have become obsessed with thinking that he will never be able to urinate on his own again.

For the first few days he wasn't able to breathe well, even with the breathing tube in his mouth, so they had laid him on his stomach, 'prone'. His arms were raised so his hands lay either side of his head. His nappy was on back to front so it could be easily changed by the nurses. He was otherwise naked. His body was very cold and pale because they kept him deliberately chilled to prevent further bleeding, swelling of the brain or infection.

Today, though, they are able to turn him over so he can lie on his back. Because he has been lying on his front for so long, his eyelids and cheeks are swollen. Added to that, they have placed electrodes on his head for an EEG and have covered them with a white knitted cap. The breathing tube is in his mouth, and another tube is taped to his cheek and going up his nose, delivering fluids. He is unrecognisable.

Everything Changes

22 February 2012

The EEG they performed yesterday doesn't tell them anything at all. So they do an MRI. It shows Evan has massive damage across the bilateral plates of his brain. His organs haven't suffered any damage.

That's all I know. I don't seek any further information from the doctors, and no one approaches me with more. I am a naturally curious person, but in these times I realise that every question I ask has an awful answer. My self-preservation instinct screams 'Shut up!' every time a doctor walks into the room. Every now and then a well-meaning friend will ask a medic a question and I hate them for it, in case the answer is too much for me to bear.

A haematologist arrives this afternoon to discuss whether the bleeding on the brain might be caused by haemophilia. After a thorough conversation regarding Evan's medical history she decides to rule it out.

I tell her about my issues with the neurologist. It has become a frequent talking point, probably because I am beginning to like the affirmation that the other doctors are giving me (since I am not getting much positivity on anything else). She does not disappoint, and says she will speak to her.

'It doesn't serve this hospital well if our patients or their parents feel they are being poorly treated.'

This makes me feel a little better, like I have just a tiny little bit of control in all of this mess.

Later, though, I find the neurologist at Evan's bedside. I tell

45

her to apologise to Evan for the way she dismissed his chances of survival.

'I'm not going to apologise for doing my job,' she says.

'It's not your job to give your opinion if it's not properly formed.'

'I think you misconstrued what I said.'

'It's your job to make sure I don't misconstrue. This is my son. He is the most important thing to me. And you just come along with your purse on your shoulder like you're off for a nice lunch and you give me that news and then you walk away as if you just told me what the time is.'

'You just don't like what I told you. It's very grim.'

I would like to write that I manage to use all my legal prowess and litigation skills to bat right back at her, but I don't. Instead I revert to something out of high school, screaming and shouting at her. The noise of the machines keeping Evan alive drowns out most of it, but it isn't eloquent.

Eventually, 'You can't touch him' is my best line.

'Fine, I am taking myself off the case,' she says, and walks out.

Once she is gone, and a new doctor has taken over and examined Evan, I leave the room, too. I find a place to hide, behind a soft-drinks machine in the parents' area. I squeeze myself into the space and cry. It feels like the worst moment of my life. Again.

When I finally come back towards Evan's room, a young pastor called Joel meets me at the door and starts talking to me. I am still crying – openly, freely, as I have been doing for days now, it feels. There is something about Joel that makes me want to tell him everything that is making me so deeply, horrifically despairing in this moment.

'I was happy. It was the happiest I have ever been.'

Joel stands and listens, asks some thoughtful questions, and then comes into Evan's room and says a prayer for him. By the time he says goodbye I have calmed and can muster new strength for Evan.

Jackie and Deborah bring me an early dinner and as we eat together I tell them about my spat with the neurologist. Shocked and annoyed, they start calling her 'Dr Grim'. It provides some light relief. And the name sticks.

Dr Brown has continued to visit us, sometimes asking questions and other times just chatting. She is a lively lady, strong, smart and well dressed.

I see a friend talking to her at one point. He comes over later and says to me, 'You need to throw the babysitter in front of the bus – if they can't pin this on her they will try and pin it on you. Tell them you were suspicious – tell them things she did that you didn't like.'

I can see his point, and know that he is very concerned and trying to help me. But I hadn't felt suspicious and, until now, there has been very little about Norma that I haven't liked. I decide to nip the issue in the bud. Dr Brown is walking towards the elevators at this point, so I call her over to us. I explain what my friend's concerns are, and then I tell her what my position is.

'We don't know what happened yet. There may be another explanation. If it is Shaken Baby Syndrome, then it was either Norma or it was someone she was with, but either way, she is responsible, and that's an awful thing for anyone to live with. If she did it, then it was either deliberate or it was accidental. If it was accidental, then I can forgive her. If it was deliberate, I will find a way to forgive her, and let the police take care of the rest of it. All I can do is look after Evan, and give him love and be positive around him. But I can't do that if I feel anger, I just can't. And I can't say I was suspicious because I wasn't.'

At the end of all this, Dr Brown looks at my friend and says, 'I think she has made her case.'

I know there are many people around me who feel anger at what has happened. Before I had Evan I would have felt that, too. In fact, I recall a mental image I always used to carry with me. It was my reaction should anyone hurt someone I love: feisty, aggressive, attacking. Now that I am a mother it's entirely different. My instincts simply say 'protect'. My mental image has become one of me holding Evan close, crouching over him, protecting him with my body.

On a more cerebral level, I know I need all of my energy for Evan. It is taking all I have to keep it together, and to give Evan everything I can. I am sure Evan can still sense me, and if he can, he can sense my mood. So I know that, just as I have asked visitors to hide their tears and sympathy, I have to leave my own negative energy behind if I possibly can. Evan has to have a positive environment, I am certain of that. I tell Jackie, Deborah and Liz and they will spread the word that there is to be no talking about Norma in front of me or in front of Evan, and there is otherwise to be as little negativity as possible. Friends and family will feel what they feel, and I can't change that but

Evan and I can't afford to burn any of our energy in trying to field off other people's anger.

More friends visit today, as they have continued to do so for days now. People bring their own personal tales of hope. A girl I haven't see for five years or so – since the days when I lived in Queens – shows up today and reminds me that she had been in a coma for five weeks, ten years ago.

'They said I wouldn't make it, they said I would be brain-damaged, they said my life was over. None of it came true,' she tells me.

Another friend tells me she was in a car accident when she was sixteen. As she was wheeled into ER, she could hear a doctor overhead saying, 'She's not going to make it.' She tells me it took her eight years to get back to normal. I've never known either of them as anything other than happy and successful.

23 February 2012

I wake to be reminded once again of the sheer hell life has become. There is no other way to describe it. I wish, with everything I have, that I had been the one to be injured. I would gladly take all of this from Evan if only I could. Instead, though, my beautiful boy, the little baby I love with everything I have, is lying in a coma in a hospital bed, with machines keeping him alive. I don't know if he will ever wake up, if he will ever eat or breathe on his own. I don't have any idea whether this hell will improve or get worse. I wonder, with a spike of anxiety, if I will look back on these days as our last days together or if I will remember them as the darkness before things got better.

I meet with Detective Reyes and Dr Brown, separately. It is draining. It has been a day or two since I've had to revisit what happened, and it suddenly becomes very painful to talk about it. Once they have both left, I go back and lie down on the pull-out bed next to Evan's and sleep for an hour or so. I still haven't managed more than two hours' sleep each night.

The one positive about today is that, when I raise Evan's hand to his forehead, his head moves, ever so slightly.

I miss you, Evan, so very much. My arms actually ache with emptiness.

24 February 2012

The doctors come by on 'rounds' each morning between 9am and 11am. The 'attending' holds court, while five or six residents gather round. One of the residents 'presents' to the others by doing a run-through of what is going on with each particular patient. The attending makes corrections, asks questions and gives pointers to the group.

You can see them – the doctors and students – congregating a few rooms ahead of ours. I take that as my cue to go and have a shower. It is too difficult to have to stand and listen to them discuss my son in very clinical terms, as they invite me to do each day. But to stay inside the room while they discuss Evan just outside our door is even worse, hearing only loose and occasional terms, none of which sound good. Even more frightening is the wait as the doctor walks in, sanitises her hands, examines Evan in silence and then looks up to say what she sees. I really can't take the anticipation. If they need to talk with me they can work out how to find me, but in the meantime, it is better for me to not be around for those moments.

Aside from that, though, a new nurse came on today and realised that Evan's catheter was the wrong size, so she removed it. Evan can urinate fine on his own so they didn't replace it. I think I can probably let go of my fear that Evan's hands will never grow bigger than the size they are right now, just because his fingernails haven't grown in a week.

My lovely friend (and Evan's godmother) Violet arrives from Ireland (she had moved back there from New York a few years ago). I called her on the first day and almost immediately she had a flight booked to come and see us. She has a job and two kids, so she can only manage for the weekend. It is wonderful to see my co-pilot again.

We chat for a while. I've had many lively conversations this week. Sometimes I can't stop talking at all, about anything and everything. I think it's the adrenaline. It's not really me talking. And it feels inappropriate sometimes, but I can't help it. After talking non-stop to Violet for a few hours I say, 'I hope you don't think because I'm okay right now that you've come all this way for nothing.'

'I know you're not okay, Elise,' she says.

25 February 2012

My sister Anne arrives from England. When she sees Evan, lifeless and connected to machines, she can't stop crying. I don't have the heart to tell her to stop.

The attending doctor for the day asks to see me in the green room. I tell him I am not up for it, that there is only so much I can bear to hear.

He says, 'It behoves you to talk to me.'

'It behoves you or it behoves me?'

We go to the green room anyway. Violet and Anne stay with Evan. The doctor explains that he isn't happy with Evan's breathing – it isn't showing signs of improvement. The breathing tube in his mouth is a temporary solution, but if I want to move him, especially if I want to be able to hold him, I should allow him to have a tracheotomy operation so the ventilator can be attached to a tube inserted into his neck. Apparently that is the only way he will be allowed to leave the ICU.

Then he tells me that Evan should also get a gastrointestinal feeding tube inserted directly into his abdomen. Right now he is fed baby formula through a tube in his nose that goes down the back of his throat and into his stomach. Over time, the tube could wear away the sinus, apparently. If we do the two surgeries required by each device, we will be able to move Evan to a rehabilitation hospital and get him some physical therapies.

It has been over a week since I have been able to hold Evan in my arms and I really miss that. All I can do right now is give him 'hand-hugs', by covering his little bare chest with both hands, so he can feel me. But the thought of him being operated on and being kitted out with these devices that seem so much more permanent – I can hardly stand it. Violet tries to make me feel better about the meeting: 'It's your choice. You don't need to listen to the doctor. If he was any good he'd get more than just the Saturday shifts,' she says, smiling.

I have my reservations about the procedures. I am worried about the surgeries involved, but that's not all. The ability to go to a rehab hospital is obviously a good step forward but – incredibly, really – I realise that I am scared of leaving the ICU. Better the devil you know, and all that. I don't know what things will be like in rehab. But we can't live here for ever: I'm going to say yes to both procedures.

Jackie brings chicken for dinner tonight and about ten of us pull the tables together in the parents' area and share the food. I try to be sociable for a while, but eventually the emotions win me over again and I end up sobbing uncontrollably. Violet and Anne take me back to Evan's room and then everyone leaves me in peace. I sit with Evan for a long time, and cry silently.

Later, a respiration therapist comes in to check on Evan's vent. She asks if I am okay. I tell her the doctor is not happy with Evan's breathing. She laughs out loud and says, 'It's not up to him, it's up to God!'

26 February 2012

That cry last night did me good. It cleared my head a bit.

Anne and Violet are staying in my apartment. They are both

warm and generous souls. I can imagine them fighting over who gets the bed and who gets the couch. 'No, you take the bed, I'm not that tired.' 'No, you…' and both of them ending up sleeping on the floor.

Evan's ventilator settings have been increased as he is not adding his own breaths to the limited number per minute the vent gives him. He has a bandage around his thumb that glows red. It's called a pulse-ox (pulse oximeter) and is connected to a screen that reads his pulse and oxygen levels (God only knows how). These are known as his 'saturation' levels, or 'sats' as they're commonly called in the hospital. The doctors would like his oxygen levels to be between 90 and 100 per cent, but sometimes they drop below. This is known as 'desatting', or just 'dropping his sats'. Because they have dropped quite frequently, the vent rate has been increased from 18 to 20 breaths per minute (BPM). The nurse says it is not unusual to go up and down on the vent settings like this.

A common reason for Evan dropping sats is when there is a build-up of secretions in his throat or further down, in his trachea. This is caused by the fact that his mouth and tongue don't work at all right now, and he can't swallow. Nor can he cough. So the secretions have nothing to do but sit and wait to be drawn out by the nurse (who pushes a thin catheter down his breathing tube and suctions them out) or grow in size and clog the trachea, preventing the flow of oxygen and leading to the pulse-ox alarming.

If there is a block or if Evan is desatting for some other reason, they take him off the ventilator and attach a plastic American football-shaped bag to the breathing tube (this is called an 'Ambu bag'). They pump the football part and this gives larger breaths to Evan than the vent does. It might help to shift some mucous or it might just help to get his sats back to between 90 and 100 per cent. Once it does its job, Evan goes back on the vent.

It's a terrifying process. All I can do is watch. I never know if everything is going to be okay. I can't read the nurses – they all keep the same expressionless face on while they work on him.

The genetics doctor stopped by late in the afternoon and told me they have ruled out a genetic cause. That was the last alternative they were pursuing. The diagnosis is now officially Shaken Baby Syndrome.

I just can't understand it. It is too awful for words. Could Norma really do something like that? Could I really have been so wrong about her?

27 February 2012

Every morning at around 6am a nice young man comes in and places a lead blanket over me, trying not to wake me (he always does) and then takes an X-ray of Evan to make sure his breathing and feeding tubes are sitting in the right places.

In the last few days a music therapist called Kate has been coming to visit Evan. She sings to him and plays the guitar. She takes requests, which come from me, obviously. If she doesn't know a song that I want her to play, she learns it for the next day. Today she sang 'The Evan Song'. I made this up in our happy time and I used to sing it to Evan at every opportunity. It's sung (loosely) to the tune of the song that starts, 'Hello Mudda, Hello Fadda, I am calling, from Camp Grenada':

> Your name is Evan
> It's not Kevin
> It's not Pat Nevin
> Or Aneurin Bevan
> It's not Brenda Blethyn
> This is doing my head in
> Oh Evan, Evan, Evan, Evan, Evan, cha cha cha

> Your middle name is Louis
> It's not Pooey
> It's not Kung fooey
> It's not Bambooey
> It isn't Hughie
> Nor is it Duwie
> Oh Louis, Louis, Louis, Louis, Louis, cha cha cha.

The song has no particular meaning, and it is made up of entirely incongruous references, which are chosen only because they rhyme with each other. I sing along, too, or not, depending on how teary I feel at any given time.

23 February 2012

I slept next to Evan in his bed last night. The nurse said it would be safe. I fought sleep for as long as I could, inhaling as much of Evan as possible. When Anne came in this morning I was still asleep. She said my forehead was touching Evan's.

Dr Baird is the attending physician this week. He is an older gentleman with a full head of white hair, dark-rimmed glasses and a fondness for flannel shirts. He looks like the type to take holidays in Vermont in the winter and Martha's Vineyard in the summer. He is nicer and warmer than other doctors we have met. Nonetheless, I still fear his morning visits.

He comes in to talk to me today, along with a resident doctor, who introduces herself as Dr Lisa. We don't get far into a conversation before I start crying. Dr Lisa puts her arm around me and they both listen as I explain the fear I feel when they come around each morning. She says I shouldn't fear them because they are here to help.

This has a hollow ring to it. If Evan needed his appendix out or a Band-Aid then it would be a great point, but, as they very well know, there is not a thing they can do to help us right now.

Dr Baird, though, steps in and is very comforting. He tells me that I have an impressive amount of support. 'Every time I look in here there's a bunch of people with you.'

Then he tells me, 'What some parents like to do is to set aside a "perspective date". Just pick a date, one far out, say, 4 July, and just aim for it. You could say you want to be in rehab by then, or maybe you want to be home. Or don't have any particular goal, just keep that date in your sights.'

That makes sense. It is also reassuring to hear a doctor talk about Evan in the longer term. It makes me realise that it has been a long time since I have heard anyone talk about Evan dying.

29 February 2012

Last night I dreamt Evan was a hamburger and someone ate a chunk out of him, making my job (of getting him better) even harder. When I woke up next to him and realised things weren't that bad, I actually felt relief.

It didn't last long. I was a mess all day today. These last two weeks of shock and anxiety and fear and grief, combined with the effort to stay positive as well as to be sociable with all the visitors – all of it suddenly seemed to come crashing together into a fireball of raw emotions that I just couldn't handle any more. My anxiety levels went through the roof. Every time there was any kind of ventilator issue I had to leave the room in a panic. I told Anne, 'I need help.' I've never said that to anyone before in my life. I called my doctor and was prescribed anti-depressants and an anti-anxiety medication called Ativan. Jackie collected the prescription for me, and she and Deborah met Anne and me for lunch.

Deborah has done some research about anxiety and can report having read somewhere that no one ever falls apart in a crisis, but now that the high drama is over and things have settled, my brain, still being on high alert, has nothing to bounce around and so the neurons (or whatever they are) are now free floating, generating and enjoying the anxiety that I haven't had time to indulge in up until now.

The Ativan certainly helps and I feel much calmer. Then come the floods of tears again. Anne takes me back to Evan's room. She is just as emotional a person as I am and the two of us sit crying, stopping, crying again, setting the other one off. Joel walks in as we both sit there in a heap of sobs. He sits with us for a while, saying nothing phenomenal or extraordinary, but somehow manages to get us both to a better place.

'I walked into this room and I just felt helpless,' he says, 'Is that how you feel?'

This lets Anne and I talk about all the things that we really do feel helpless about. It lets us flush out some issues that are not problems at all. I tell her that I worry that I won't ever be able to go to Scotland and see our mum again. She immediately says that she can easily come and look after Evan so I can travel home. This alone removes a whole vein of anxiety from me. Then Anne says she can't stand to see me so upset. I tell her that crying like this is a good thing, that it actually helps me. This makes her feel better, too. Joel says another prayer over Evan and then leaves us, in much better shape than he had found us.

I March 2012

Today isn't bad, and this evening Anne and I have dinner in a local café. I come back to Evan's room to begin my now nightly routine – make the bed, get changed into clothes that don't look like pyjamas but which are comfortable enough to sleep in, walk across the ICU to the parents' shower room and wash in cold water (that's all there is in the parents' bathroom in the evening), come back and then clamber up into Evan's bed.

In the middle of my preparations tonight, Dr Lisa stops by our room 'for a chat' (she says). Her timing seems a little off – it is almost midnight – but we sit down on the chairs to the side of Evan's bed. She wants to know if I am 'realistic' about Evan. It catches me off guard, but I tell her what I know she wants to hear, balanced with what I can stomach, saying: 'I know that the MRI is bad, but no one knows where that will go. I know we have months, if not years, of rehab.'

She says, 'You know he might never breathe on his own. Kids on vents are in and out of hospital.'

'Where are you going with this?' I ask.

'Well, there are other options. Many parents with a child like this decide that it isn't fair to continue and opt to withdraw care.'

I am not fooled by the euphemism. She is asking me if I want to switch off the machines that keep my beloved Evan alive.

'That's my son,' I say, pointing to Evan. 'I believe in him and I believe he can get better. That's his picture up there on the wall,' I say, pointing to a photograph of Evan from a month ago. In it, he is sitting in his little chair, wearing only a nappy, with puréed carrots dripping from his mouth down his chest, his massive blue eyes staring out.

'I look at that picture and I see Evan and I know that is the same little boy as is lying in that bed. I will never give up on him.'

Then I tell her about a dream I once had. It was a year or so before I became pregnant with Evan. I had been trying for only a few months but was getting impatient. The dream wasn't really a dream, it was some kind of visitation. A boy – probably eighteen or so – sat on the edge of my bed. He was beautiful. He had golden blond hair, short and swept forward, and the most alert eyes. When I woke up, I could hear two people talking in my head.

'No, not Kevin...' they were saying.

Evan, I thought. That young man was Evan. I had chosen the name when I had first thought of having children. Evans is my mother's maiden name and so Evan seemed to be a perfect fit. And sure enough, in Evan's first few days of life, I could see that beautiful young man's face in his.

'And he didn't have any machines attached to him,' I tell Dr Lisa.

She asks a few more questions, but it is a courteous and civil exchange and she doesn't force the issue, even adding, as she leaves the room, 'Well, now I believe in him, too.' We smile as we say goodnight. Then I crawl into bed next to Evan and lie awake and troubled all night long.

2 March 2012

Tonight Anne and I talked a bit about what it would be like if Evan remains severely disabled.

'All I want is for his little eyes to see us and show us that he knows we love him,' she tells me.

I've felt this all week, but it is lovely to hear her say it, too.

Of course I want more for him, but I will love him with all I have, no matter what. It would make a world of difference, though, if I could see some indication that he knows how much I love him. Right now, we are such a long way away from any of that. When the doctors open Evan's eyelids, his eyes don't move at all. The pupils don't react. Even when he is being moved around, you can see that his eyeballs just stay exactly where they are.

3 March 2012

Evan's six-month birthday.

I have been reporting each and every little twitch Evan makes to the medics as and when they happen (which isn't really all that often). It has become apparent, though, that what I see as, at least, tiny improvements are making no impression on the doctors or nurses at all. In fact, I'm starting to believe they think I'm going a little crazy. Dr Baird comes in on his final day of rounds today. I tell him that I have seen Evan's head move on its own, without anyone touching him.

'That would be interesting,' he says. As in, 'if it were verified by one of us'.

I probably am going a bit crazy. I am so focused on looking for tiny movements from Evan that when I am in the washroom today I stare at the trash can so hard that I actually believe it moves.

Before he leaves, Dr Baird examines Evan then turns to me as he is leaving the room and says, warmly, 'Well, nothing new medically, I'm afraid, but keep observing him and let us know what you see.'

Friends arrive with cake and drinks and toast Evan. For the most part, though, I sit in the corner sobbing as everyone else stands awkwardly around.

Everything Changes

Violet has teamed up with my friend Stacy, who tells me today that together they have made a website all about Evan. There are pictures of him when he was well, and a brief description of his condition now. There is also an option – if people want – to make a donation.

'People want to help you, Elise, and sometimes money is the only practical way,' Violet tells me when we speak on the phone later.

I am touched, but I feel quite uncomfortable at the idea of charity. I don't want to make Violet or Stacy feel bad, so I decide to let the issue lie for a while. The website isn't live yet anyway.

4 March 2012

Evan and I have a good day today. After telling Dr Baird yesterday that Evan moves on his own, he does it again today with a nurse as a witness. A new doctor is attending and when she comes into our room, the nurse reports it, very seriously and professionally. I want to high-five them both. The doctor says that we should expect some improvement at this stage, but to be aware that any improvement is bound to be slow. But, she adds, it is always good to have hope. I love this doctor. Maybe she just hasn't read enough of Evan's file yet, but being told by a doctor to keep hope alive is a rarity around here.

I Believe in Evan

5 March 2012

I wake up feeling a little low, but otherwise okay. Today's nurse is quite chatty. I ask her if she has children.

'Yes,' she says, 'Two. They are both great. My husband and I are really lucky. Actually, I'm pregnant again, just three months.'

Then she looks at Evan and back at me and starts to cry.

'I'm sorry,' she says, 'I don't mean to cry in front of you but I just think this is so sad.'

Thanks, lady.

The nurse leaves the room and Music Therapy Kate walks in right on cue.

'You look like you're really going through it right now,' she says to me with a consoling chuckle.

She has learned a song that I had asked her to play for Evan, Sade's 'By Your Side'. I've been playing it for him since his first days, when I brought him home from the hospital. It's a lovely soothing song: 'Do you think I would leave your side, babe? You know me better than that...'

Kate sings it beautifully, lightly strumming her guitar. It lifts my spirits and I almost forget the nurse's tears.

Then three doctors in white coats walk in and introduce themselves as rehabilitation specialists. Dr Kim, an energetic Asian lady, does all the talking.

'Get him to rehab, see what he can do, and then when you get home, bring him to me for follow-up.'

She is full of positivity.

'Evan, Evan, wake up Evan!' she chirps.

He, of course, doesn't respond. She looks him over and says, in a cheery tone, 'Well, the good thing is that the outcome doesn't always match the picture (referring to the MRI).'

After this, the hospital social worker, Soulemar, comes in with pamphlets from two rehab centres, Blythedale Children's Hospital in Westchester, just above Yonkers, and New Jersey's Children's Specialized Hospital. She tells me to think about which one I would like Evan to go to. It feels like things are improving at last.

Later, I go out into the waiting area where the phone reception is much better (it is very poor in Evan's room) and try to call my mum to let her know about the morning's events. As the signal on my phone improves, I see that I have several voice messages. I listen to them. One is from Ms Dominique from ACS, asking me to call her. The message is from Friday and is now three days old.

I start to look for Ms Dominique's number when my phone rings. She is calling me. I try to explain that I only just got her message, but she cuts me off: 'There was a child safety conference at our office this morning and you and the babysitter were supposed to be there.'

'I only just heard your message from last week,' I explain, 'but even if I had received it then, I couldn't have gone. I don't leave Evan's bedside and I really do not want to be in the same room as the babysitter.'

'I have to tell you this, so please listen carefully,' she tells me. 'There is a scheduled appearance in Family Court at 2pm today. ACS is petitioning to have Evan removed from your custody.'

I can hardly draw a breath. I hadn't seen this coming, not in a million years.

'How can you do this to me?' I manage to say.

'It wasn't my decision,' she says, sounding uncomfortable.

It is already 1pm at this point. I call my good friend Randi Karmel, who is also a matrimonial and family lawyer. She has already been to visit us at the hospital several times and knows what is going on. I tell her as much as I can about the phone call.

'Meet me at court at a quarter to two,' she says and then hangs up.

Deborah walks into our room with a cup of coffee for me. I stare at her, with the phone still in my hand.

Within ten minutes the two of us are in a cab going all the way down town to the courthouses. Pauline happens to call and I explain it to her as much as I can, adding, 'I can't believe this situation just got even worse.'

I also call Liz, who works near the court, and ask her to meet us there. Deborah calls Jackie and lets her know what is going on. Jackie drops whatever it is she is doing and goes directly to the hospital to sit with Evan while I am gone.

We find the floor the courtroom is on. Randi is already there. She is standing in the hallway talking animatedly with a young man with dark hair and a grey suit, and a young blonde female. They are both lawyers. One is the attorney for ACS, Jesse Lubin. He is short and very young looking. The Legal Aid attorney, Jennifer Weaver, doesn't look much older. She, apparently, has been appointed Evan's lawyer.

'Sit over there. I will be with you in a minute,' Randi tells me, pointing at the row of benches in the hallway of the courtrooms. She isn't smiling.

By this point Liz has arrived. She and Deborah sit either side of me. I sit with my head in my hands, sobbing. I keep saying over and over, 'Please don't let them separate us.' I know that neither Evan nor I will fare well if we aren't together. The only good I can do for him is to be by his side at all times, and here is this massive threat that I won't be able to do even that.

The threat of losing him is what drove me to be a single mother. The reason I attended all those doctors' appointments alone, without a partner or even so much as a known sperm donor. I did all that because I couldn't bear the thought that someone might one day try and take Evan away from me, even just for a moment. And here I am.

Randi comes over to me.

'You have a fight on your hands,' she tells me. 'I can't talk them out of this action.'

We are called into court. I am crying inconsolably. The judge seems cranky and irritable towards each attorney in equal measure. Randi does her very best, telling the judge that the NYPD view me only as a victim, that the babysitter is their suspect and she hasn't been named on the ACS petition; that this is the longest I have been away from Evan's bedside, that I love him and couldn't possibly hurt him and that it would be a gross injustice to separate us.

The judge responds, 'There is nothing about what the mother is doing that I am going to interfere with.'

He leaves me with full access and decision-making authority

over Evan but probably to protect himself as much as anyone, grants a legal remand of Evan to the custody of the state. It is an easy decision for the judge as Evan is confined to a hospital bed for the foreseeable future with no immediate prospect of me taking him home anyway. It won't have any impact whatsoever on anything, and it doesn't affect my role with Evan in any way. Humiliating and harsh on me, for sure, but not damaging to Evan, which is all that matters.

A new court date is calendared for April, and a trial date scheduled for the end of October. I sit crying throughout the hearing. I've never cried openly in court before. I've never worn hiking trousers and a man-size purple T-shirt in court before either, but these were the only clean clothes I could find at the hospital today.

Once it is over, Deborah, Liz and I race downstairs, jump in another cab, and ask the driver to take us back to Columbia Hospital as quickly as possible. I want to be back with my boy. On the journey, Soulemar calls me and tells me she is appalled that ACS has done this to me.

When we arrive at the ICU, we tell Jackie everything that happened. Then the four of us sit around Evan, trying to decompress the events of the day.

6 March 2012

Jackie calls to say Detective Reyes has called her because she couldn't get through to me. She told Jackie to tell me that the NYPD is furious with ACS for bringing the petition against me.

'This is not the direction we are going in at all – Elise is a victim here too.'

Detective Reyes also said that ACS and the NYPD are supposed to decide when to act together and that she is angry that ACS acted without them.

This makes me feel quite a bit better, although the sting of yesterday hasn't left me yet.

Around lunchtime, the Indian neurologist – with the satchel – who had been with Dr Grim that first full day, shows up with two neurology residents. Almost as soon as they enter the room he spills the entire contents of his satchel on the floor. 'A neurologist's lunch,' he says (whatever that means), as he picks everything up. Then he asks me whether I mind if they do some tests on Evan.

I say I don't, so they set to, calling Evan's name, pinching him in various places, observing the heart monitor as they do so. There is no significant response from him to any of this, and I know it.

The neurologist turns to me and asks me if I am realistic about the future. As with Dr Lisa, I tell him exactly what he wants to hear ('months, if not years, etc, etc.').

Then he says, 'Well, there are some options available, depending on your personal ethics and morals…'

'I've had this discussion already and the answer is no,' I say, stopping him mid-flow.

He has the decency to apologise, and says he didn't realise I had already been asked about 'withdrawing care'. I ask him to spread the word among the other doctors, and that I am not to be asked again. He nods. Then all three leave.

I climbed into bed and hand-hug Evan.

Later, Dr Brown shows up, looking very concerned. She asks me about the court hearing.

'It was awful,' I tell her.

'I'm sure it was,' she replies.

Like Detective Reyes, she says she is very annoyed at ACS.

Jackie comes in and the three of us start talking about Evan's upcoming procedures and the various rehabilitation facilities that are available. Dr Brown seems happy to just shoot the breeze for a little while. It gradually takes my mind away from the events of lunchtime and the day before.

The sun is setting over New Jersey by now and the light in the room is starting to fade. Dr Brown gathers her things to leave. As she is doing so, the week's attending doctor comes in. He is middle-aged, with greying hair and a reddish complexion, which is accentuated by his salmon-coloured shirt.

'When is Evan's operation going to be?' I ask him, referring to the tracheotomy and G-tube procedures.

'Well, we should all sit down and talk about what's going on,' he says.

Oh, not again.

'Look,' I say, 'I've had the conversation twice already and I won't withdraw care. I would withdraw it from myself before I withdrew it from Evan.'

He tries to persuade me anyway. I interrupt him and say, 'With respect, you are going to walk out of here at the end of this week and I am never going to see you again. So I'm not going to listen to you try and change my mind about a situation I have already made a decision on.'

He looks a bit annoyed and then says, 'Well, if you are convinced then we might as well go ahead with the surgery.'

'Right. When?' I ask, a little impatiently.

'Look,' he says, suddenly becoming animated, and doing a semi-dance towards Evan, 'he's about as brain dead as you can be without being brain dead. He has no feeling in his face. When we move him, his heart rate is supposed to jump around and it doesn't. He'll probably never breathe on his own. That's about as good as you're going to get.'

As his use of the word 'that', referring to Evan, lying there, rings through me, the doctor draws breath, ready to continue.

'Are you done?' I cut in. 'Because it sounds like you are going to start from the beginning and say that all over again and I don't think there's any need.'

'Okay,' he says. 'Any questions?'

'Yes,' I say, 'When is the operation?'

He rolls his eyes and starts pacing the floor again, then he says, 'Maybe Friday.'

For a second he stares coldly at me and then adds, 'But where are you going to send him? He can't stay here.'

As if I'd want him to after all of this.

'We're going to go to Blythedale,' I say, suddenly (randomly) deciding that is the rehab place for us.

'But Blythedale won't take hopeless cases. He might go somewhere else, but he won't go there,' he shoots back.

I allow an awkward silence to descend and eventually he leaves the room. I sense his disappointment that he hasn't persuaded me. I don't know if he senses my agony.

I see Jackie and Dr Brown look at each other. I can tell they are shocked.

Once again, I climb into bed with Evan. Jackie and Dr Brown leave the room, giving me some privacy.

My mind is blank, as I lie there next to Evan, hanging on to his little cold body.

After some time, Jackie comes back in with a sandwich for me. She asks me how I am. I can barely speak. She asks me if I want her to stay; I don't.

'Liz is outside,' she tells me. I nod.

'Don't cut us off,' she adds, before she leaves.

After a while I go out to Liz and tell her I can't talk right now. She nods, but makes no signs of leaving. Instead she says, 'Well, I'll be here if you need me, but if you don't, that's okay too.'

I go back to Evan's room, lie on the pull-out bed and stare at the ceiling. The attending doctor comes back in at one point and says, 'You know, I didn't mean to be harsh there, I just want you to be realistic. If you have any questions, let me know.'

I stare at him. I am not going to say anything that might make him feel better about what he has just done to me. He leaves.

I lie there some more, trying to make sense of the jangled mess that is inside my head. It feels like I have been knocked off my already shaky ladder, and am free-falling with absolutely nothing to cling to. I need something to grab a hold of, desperately.

I think of the dream – of Evan as a young man, alert and perfect, on the edge of my bed. I have thought of it a million times in these past few weeks, wondering if it can be trusted. Tonight I have to immerse myself in the hope that it can, that somehow this damaged boy can become that beautiful young man, with not a blemish on him, inside or out.

I remember Stephanie in Woodstock, and what she said to me: 'Do not listen to the devils.'

I have absolutely no doubt that withdrawing care is not the right thing to do. I can feel that in my core. But it's not easy to stand firm in the face of three different, and increasingly strong, forces. Of course, you can't rely on any psychic reading for something as important as a decision about your child's health and survival. I am still painfully aware that Evan might well remain in a vegetative state for the rest of his life but I am equally aware that, if this is the case, it is our path together. 'Withdrawing care' has never even seemed like a 'decision' that was there to be made. I intuitively know not to agree to it, and I also know that it is my role in life to live with the consequences, no matter what.

But my will must remain strong until we get the operations done on Friday.

I start to paint the devils. Dr Lisa, the Indian neurologist with the satchel, and today's attending doctor become three levels of devil. Lisa is a small devil, without much sting, easily swatted away. The neurologist has more power because he has more experience, but he doesn't hold up against much resistance either. The attending doctor, however, with his reddish skin tone, bulbous nose, and deep pink shirt is easy to imagine as a very angry devil. He has horns and a tail, angrily swishing around as he stomps the floor of Evan's room. But I overcome him too. I send him away to blow off his own steam. I rename him Dr Evil. It makes me feel like I have a little control.

I think about my dad. A week before he died a nurse told me he had an aortic tear. 'It might be days, weeks or years,' she said, 'but that rupturing is what is going to kill him.' She was wrong: Dad died of pneumonia. A hollow victory, I know, but they can be wrong; they can.

I start to think about impossible situations I've been in before. Coming to America with $700 in my pocket and surviving anyway; becoming a lawyer; getting pregnant after sixteen months of trying; feeling okay about being gay; starting my own practice without any real money behind me. All of these things seemed too far out of reach to even contemplate at one point. And then, of course, there were plenty of law cases to draw from – cases where I didn't seem to stand a chance at the outset, but somehow managed to win anyway.

Running, that is another good example to focus on. I used to run short distances. Then I went through a rotten break-up with a girlfriend and, to distract myself, I signed up for a half-marathon two weeks before it was to take place. I had never run that distance before and I couldn't possibly train properly in that time. As I ran the first mile of the race I started to panic. 'I can't do this,' I thought, as people ran noisily past me along the wooden boardwalk of Coney Island. Then I realised how stupid I was being: of course I could run the first mile. Then I ran the second, and on it went, mile by mile. By mile twelve, when I was starting to hurt, I started saying over and over again, 'I am Elise

Schwarz, and I can do anything.' I completed the race. I have run a dozen or more half-marathons since, as well as one full one.

Buoyed by these thoughts, I start to let all the anthems of hope I can imagine sing out inside my head, in a garbled, jangling jumble.

When you walk through the storm hold your head up high
Keep right on to the end of the road
And don't be afraid of the rain
Tie yourself to the mast my friend and the storm will end
At the end of the storm is a golden sky, and the sweet silver song of the lark.
There was a soldier, a Scottish soldier
If you think I would leave your side babe, you know me better than that
You'll NEVER WALK ALONE.

I let each line wring out in my head, pumping me up, word by word, from the flattened mess Dr Evil has left me in.

By the time I am through with all of this I am back on my ladder, galvanised in the moment, knowing that now is the time to get galvanised for the future ahead.

I go out to Liz who, sure enough, is waiting (for several hours at this point) in the waiting area, and I present her with a list of work files that I need help to organise for the purpose of offloading to another lawyer.

'I'm giving it all up and I'm going to concentrate full-time on getting Evan better.'

'Okay then,' she says, in her usual non-judgemental way.

And that is that.

Back in the ward, all the nurses know about my ordeal of the past few days and all are tiptoeing more than usual. When I get ready for bed the night nurse lets me hold Evan while she changes his sheets.

As I hold his limp, cold, undressed body, covered in sensors and with cords trailing, I say to him over and over again, 'I will never give up on you.'

Tonight my prayer to God is for us to get into Blythedale. If we do, there is, in fact, hope for Evan. I add, 'Dear God, I believe I am right to refuse to withdraw care. If you disagree with me on this one, please contact me directly.'

7 March 2012

Despite my resolve of last night, I wake up feeling drained. I can't even stand up at first. Dr Evil has really done a number on me. It feels like I have been through an emotional dishwasher. I know the usual term is 'rollercoaster', but they have 'ups' as well as 'downs', which my situation does not, right now. Gradually though, my day comes together. Deborah brings me coffee and a bagel. Later, Music Therapy Kate plays some positive songs for us.

I call my mum. We haven't talked in much detail about Evan's condition, but I know I have to get it out in the open with her.

'There's a chance that Evan will be severely disabled,' I tell her.

'And we'll love him just as much,' she says cheerily, and without missing a beat. Her voice has not a hint of fear in it.

It is probably not a coincidence that I get a visit from another Catholic priest today. He is an older man, a Father Johnstone, and I have seen him around before, although he has never spoken to me and he has never visited Evan. He walks in wearing the typical black suit and dog collar, but he has an over-sized pin on his lapel that urges, 'Don't take your organs to heaven – we need them here on earth.'

He talks a bit about how he has Scottish ancestors. I indulge him, though I am quite sure I know what is coming next.

'Let me tell you about some of my friends in this hospital,' he begins, suddenly getting to his point.

'There's Ryan downstairs, who is waiting for a new heart, Jimmy along the hall here, who needs a new liver. There's many of my friends here and they're just waiting for a little miracle.'

I let him talk, and say nothing in response. Eventually he runs out of steam. He leaves, without so much as a prayer for Evan. Had I not been brought up to show respect for priests I would have said aloud what I think inside, 'Get out, get out, get out, Father Johnstone! I will not let my son die. His organs are not for harvesting.'

It is also probably not a coincidence that, an hour later, the child in the room next to us is moved to a room across the floor, and in his place arrives a twelve-year-old extremely disabled girl. She writhes all day long, twisting her body, screeching and wailing. She is ventilator dependent too, and has been admitted because of a chest infection. It's clear, though, that this is the way she always is, infection or not. Perhaps I am supposed to see this girl and realise that this could be how Evan turns out too. I think about that for a while. Then I see the girl's mother. She looks calm and she looks like she cares very much for her daughter. Nothing about what I see weakens my decision. In fact, it reminds me that love can conquer all.

Pauline arrives from Spain this afternoon. I meet her at reception and we hug.

'I'm so sorry,' she keeps saying.

For once, I am in a position to be more stoic and practical than her. I soothe and calm her.

We go in to see Evan. I realise how difficult it must be for her to see him for the first time like this. Joel comes in and the three of us chat for a bit. I tell him about Dr Evil, and how I am not going to withdraw care.

'I would have supported you either way,' he says, and I know he means it.

Then Jackie comes in, full of the joys of life. She has just taken a tour of Blythedale. Each parent is supposed to go and check it out before their child is admitted, but I didn't want to leave Evan so she said she would do it. She, of course, had heard Dr Evil say Blythedale wouldn't take us. She looks so excited when she walks in that I know it is good news.

'Will they take us?' I ask.

'They said they will be delighted to take Evan,' she beams.

Finally, an 'up' – the good news we have been waiting for so long.

Almost immediately, three doctors walk in with consent

forms. Both operations are scheduled to take place in two days' time.

Pauline, Jackie and I go to the local bar and I eat food for the first time in days. I feel like I am ten feet tall. I am fully aware that a deep dip could be right around the corner, but in these unusual times I am learning to celebrate the highs as and when they come along. For tomorrow they could be gone. Again.

8 March 2012

When Music Therapy Kate comes in this morning she says, 'You look better.'

I certainly feel better. I feel defiant in the face of Dr Evil.

Dr Brown stops by to check on me again. I tell her about my newfound resolve.

'The future is unwritten,' I tell her.

'No,' she says, in her wise way, 'you are writing your own future.'

She tells Pauline and me to go out and enjoy the sunshine the day is offering and to bring back some positive energy to give to Evan, which we do. Then, this evening Pauline, Liz and I go downtown to my office and start to break it down.

I realise the magnitude of what I am doing, tearing down what I have taken five years to build up. Each file is being reassigned or boxed up and sent to storage. I lost many a night's sleep building this practice, ate cheap food; went without luxuries while it grew. I put myself through the mill for every client. I stood victorious in some courtrooms, and exhausted and beaten in others. I loved it all.

I Believe in Evan

I've been able to do a lot of dismantling of my caseload from Evan's bedside. Most clients and opposing counsel are kind when I call to tell them I have to close my practice. One client says, in the same vein as most of the others, 'The most important thing is looking after your family. I wish you all the best and will keep you in my thoughts and prayers.'

Another client isn't so nice and tries to use my withdrawal to boost his case (it doesn't work, but it does give me a headache trying to iron things out with the tribunal). Attorneys I have once sparred with express their sadness and hope for Evan. Only one attorney seeks any advantage, although this same lawyer refused to grant me an extension of time on a motion when my dad passed away. Generally, though, the words of kindness far outweigh any badness.

I have arranged to give the vast majority of my cases to another attorney who is happy to boost his practice. Other clients will find their own new counsel. I have kept one case. It is such a complex and convoluted arbitration and has been going on for so long that it wouldn't be fair on the client, or any other attorney, to step aside. It won't require any work for a few months anyway.

So, for the most part, I no longer have a law practice. I have no doubt that giving up work is the right thing to do. I am doing it entirely for Evan and there's nothing that could ever trump that. All I want is to give Evan everything I have.

Everything Changes

9 March 2012

Evan is taken to surgery at 8am. Pauline and I sit in his empty room, waiting for news. We both stare at the space his bed has left as a cleaner mops the floor. Pauline tries her best to distract me, but it's an uphill battle.

After two hours we are told that both surgeries have gone well and that the doctor is bringing Evan back to the room. When he arrives, he looks the same as when he left except for the new tubes that now run into his neck and abdomen to replace those that had run into his nose and mouth.

I am allowed to give Evan one kiss before being sent to get a coffee while the nurses settle him.

My body aches. I've been so tense for so long, but the relief of the surgery being over has allowed me to relax a bit. My muscles, now allowed a brief recess, are telling me they hate me.

10 March 2012

Now that Evan is through his surgery and all is well, I have started to obsess about the ACS case. I wish I didn't have to; I only want to think about Evan.

I looked up the ACS lawyer's credentials online. He has been an attorney for only three years. His demeanour suggests that it could be less. I have seen his type a hundred times, in the hallways of immigration courtrooms and criminal and family courts. At recruitment time the law firms pass on them and the district attorneys' offices don't want them either, so they end up in agencies like ACS, where they are promised plenty of courtroom experience in return for a very low wage. Then they learn on the job. They work at the behest of their supervisors, who know they own these lawyers. The supervisor can tell them to do anything and the lawyer has to do it. In my case, a nameless faceless supervisor has decided to bring this action against me and just see where the chips fall. As cruel and heartless as that might be, it's an easy choice for the supervisor. They won't ever get their hands dirty because they won't ever see me face-to-face.

11 March 2012

Randi calls and tells me she has heard about my conversation with Dr Evil. I tell her I want to bring a complaint against him. She tells me not to. 'You don't know who you are going to need to testify for you and it makes no sense to get on anyone's wrong side right now.'

I find this really frustrating, but I can see her point. She also says that we can't go ahead with the website Violet and Stacy set up to raise funds: it might look to the court that I am profiting from Evan's condition. I really didn't want the website to go live anyway, so it's more of a relief. I still feel stung at the vaguest of insinuations against me, though. These accusations that a few weeks ago would have sounded ridiculous now, apparently, could be real. If they can drag me away from Evan's bedside and down to court to take legal custody of him from me, they can do anything.

Pauline leaves to go back to Spain. I'm always sad to see her go, but of course this is particularly hard. She cries as we say goodbye and calls me 'an inspiration'. I don't feel inspiring; I feel tired and sad and scared, and I want Evan to wake up and smile at me. And then I want us both to go home to our warm, cosy little studio apartment and take up from where we left off.

12 March 2012

For whatever reason, doctors and nurses seem to work from the principle that it's best to remove all hope from the families of very sick patients. I am sure there are good reasons for this, and I'm sure most of them are to do with trying not to get sued, but I really feel they have got it all wrong. Trying to get through these moments – these hours that become days that become weeks – without optimism would be deadly. Hope, even without any doctor's justification for it, is the only thing that has allowed me to keep it all together.

Today Evan starts arching his back up, over and over again. It is the biggest movement I've seen him make so far, and I go out to the nurse, Jenene, and tell her about it. She barely acknowledges me and continues writing up her notes. I go back into the room but am so annoyed that I go back out and say to her, 'These things might not mean anything to you but they mean everything to me', and I walk away.

A while later, when friends have arrived, she comes into the room and says, 'Let's hug it out', and extends her arms to me.

The last thing I want to do is to hug her, but I don't want to seem churlish so I do it anyway.

13 March 2012

A very good day: the nurse wakes me up to say that Evan's pupils are now reacting to light shone into them. They weren't until now. She tells me she isn't sure what this means, but it is 'something new, medically'.

We have been here for so long that the rotation of attending doctors has returned to the first week we were here. The female doctor with the long silver hair is back. I certainly don't want to ask her any questions, as I already know her to be very negative with us.

When she shows up to examine Evan, she doesn't mention the pupils (which must mean it's a good sign or you can bet your bottom dollar she'd have jumped all over the negatives). She tells me that we are going to Blythedale on Monday. I tell her I am very pleased, and that I feel that we have outstayed our welcome. She says, 'No, not at all.' Then, for no apparent reason, she adds that when Evan goes to Blythedale, because he's on a ventilator, he will probably get pneumonia and will then be brought back to the ICU. I ignore this.

15 March 2012

A former client of mine, Ilana, has been visiting a lot. Today she brings two rabbinical students. She is Jewish and knows Evan and I are not Jewish; it doesn't matter to her. She wants to help in ways she understands. It certainly doesn't matter to me – I think it's lovely of her. The students sing a song in Hebrew, while one of them plays guitar. It is lovely to hear their deep voices. Ilana is disappointed it doesn't wake Evan up.

Dr Brown comes by. I tell her Evan is improving. He moves a little and she is very pleased. She says she has come to say goodbye to Evan and me. She tells me that she will testify at the babysitter's trial, if there is one. I ask her if she is sure it is SBS. Yes, she says, she is. I ask her if it has anything to do with Evan's first hospitalisation, in January. I know she has looked at those medical records too.

'Yes,' she says, 'There is no doubt in my mind that this was going on then too.'

I start crying. 'I'm sorry, Evan,' I keep saying over and over again.

Dr Brown puts her hand on my shoulder.

'You have to keep going, put that behind you. Focus on the future.' Then she leaves.

16 March 2012

My lovely friend Gerry (my first roommate in the USA, and with whom I shared those five wonderful years in San Francisco) shows up at the ICU today. Like Violet, he lives in Ireland now. He had heard of a conference he could register for in New York City, which would allow him to come and visit Evan and me. I am so pleased to see him. He walks in, wearing a nice black suit, pink shirt and tie, looking as handsome as ever. I am holding Evan at the time. I start crying and Gerry does too. I tell him how this happened and of course there are more tears from us both. I'm always grateful when people don't react with anger.

Gerry and I used to do almost everything together. At one point we both got jobs at the same restaurant. Gerry used to marvel at the fact we were here, a Scottish girl and an Irish guy, riding our bikes up to the Castro in San Francisco to work in an Indian restaurant. 'How bizarre is that?' he used to say.

We sit with Evan for a long time but then I have to go and get a psych evaluation for the prescription I am taking. I leave Gerry in the room with Evan. When I come back in, a half-hour later, the poor guy is sitting with his jacket off, intensely focused on Evan and looking quite stressed. It turns out that the vent fitting keeps popping off Evan's new tracheostomy tube every time he arches. The nurse is nowhere to be seen. Gerry has been sat re-attaching my son's life support machine for the last half hour. How bizarre is this?

This evening Ilana comes back to visit. Ilana talks very little. She speaks some English, but it frustrates her to try and express herself so she does it in actions. Over the last week or so she has brought me bags of groceries, including fresh fruit and a bottle of Baileys. She has brought religious artifacts and placed them around Evan's bed. She herself seems to have a kind of love/hate relationship with God. ('How can I pray to God when it is God who has done this?' she told me, almost hysterically, yesterday.) Tonight she comes back with two rabbis and tells them to get praying. Deborah, Jackie and Gerry and I stand round Evan's bed, a little incredulous, as the two rabbis read in Hebrew at a very fast pace. Once done, Ilana hands them an envelope and then all three leave.

Later, Gerry and I go to a nearby restaurant and catch up. We chat for hours. It just feels so good to have him here, a lovely source of support and affection. When he says goodbye, he adds, 'You have to understand, Elise, that we are all thinking about you both all of the time, willing Evan to get better and making sure you're okay too.'

18 March 2012

I spend a lot of today in a bad mood. Evan is still non-responsive. His pupils will dilate just ever so slightly when a light is shone in them. His eyes won't open by themselves, but now the lids have stopped shutting properly. You can see a tiny bit of the lovely blue colour of his iris, but the eyes won't move, not on their own, and not when Evan is moved. I don't know what that means, but I'm too afraid to ask. He still doesn't have much movement really, except that if you pull his arm up into a very uncomfortable position, he will squirm ever so slightly. I can watch the monitor to find out the rate of his heart beat and what his oxygen levels are, but that's the only information I can get from him right now.

I know we are leaving to go to Blythedale tomorrow and that has promise. It's a fresh start, and the beginning of Evan's rehabilitation. But change is always disconcerting, especially in this situation.

Part Three

Blythedale

19 MARCH 2012

It's the first day of spring. The trees are bare and there's still quite a chill in the air. I feel strong as we leave the ICU. It's a beautifully sunny morning and the air feels clean and fresh. Evan is rolled into the back of the ambulance on the portable bed he has been given. I clamber in behind him and take my seat against the side wall. We are driven away from the ICU, into the unknown. The driver takes a scenic route to Blythedale, up through the greenery of Westchester County, but it matters little to us, stuck in the back of the ambulance for the forty-minute drive. Without windows, I am left to navigate the dark caverns of my mind.

I Believe in Evan

When we arrive at Blythedale, Jackie and Deborah are waiting for us outside. They have driven up ahead of us, with our luggage. They are full of excitement about how new and impressive the facility is and all the nice people they have already met. The two of them have already filled Evan's crib with a ridiculously large assortment of stuffed toys in all shapes and colours and sizes. It is a wonderful welcome, but as the paramedics roll Evan into our new room, I can't help but feel overwhelmed. I keep wondering what he and I are doing here.

We are given a little time to get settled in, then a short and chipper female doctor appears at our door. She introduces herself as Evan's doctor (Dr M). She invites me to follow her into a little windowless room. It holds a round table, four chairs, and a box of Kleenex. We are joined by a tall, younger woman, who introduces herself as Evan's social worker (SW).

We start talking. They ask me to tell them what happened. I explain as much as I can through tears and stuttering diction. They are both sympathetic but with a professional air. Once I finish telling them, the SW says, 'Sorry for your loss.' I wish she hadn't. I also wish I had the strength of mind to correct her; I haven't lost him.

Dr M discusses the plasticity of the infant brain. She explains the concept that, at such a young age, when the brain hasn't yet fully developed, function lost in areas that are damaged can be replaced by function found in other areas. From this point of view, she tells me, if you have to have a severe brain injury, this is a good age to have it. She relays all this to me without making eye contact.

She tells me they will do their best, some kids respond well, others don't, and sometimes you just need more time. 'He will never be what he was, though,' she feels the need to add. 'Neither will I,' I manage.

I make it clear to both of them that I have lots of hope. Somehow, irrationally, I suppose, I feel this might affect the level of care they give Evan.

'You always have hope,' says Dr M, still without eye contact.

There is something about her tone that isn't quite what it could be when she says this.

They ask me whom I live with.

'I live alone.'

'Well, we don't really like to send a ventilated child home to just one parent. We've done it, but you'd have to prove to us you can cope.'

I don't answer them. My thoughts are conflicted between, 'Of course I can cope', and 'How am I going to cope?'

They advise me I should get a bigger apartment in preparation for Evan's eventual release. They tell me that he will need machines at home – the ventilator, the pulse-ox, the blood pressure monitor and the feeding machines – along with other equipment. And supplies. And then there will be the nurses. He will need round-the-clock care. I can't take in the full effect of all of this; I focus instead on the easy part: my apartment is too small.

After the meeting I go back to Evan. He looks different in his new crib, and his new room. Everything feels unfamiliar. I go outside to get some air, opening the floodgates as I leave the building, crying in the dark, walking to God knows where. It just all seems so unreal, so harsh. I don't understand why we have to go through this.

Once I have calmed down a little, I resolve to give myself ten days to get accustomed to things — a mini 'perspective date' — and not to freak out between now and then.

When I come back into our new room I make up my new bed. I have been given a little fold-down couch next to Evan's crib. No more sleeping in the same bed as him, there just isn't room.

20 March 2012

I slept until about 9am this morning, and woke to find a complimentary breakfast waiting for me — instant coffee and a sausage scramble that has been repeating on me all day. They only give you a free breakfast on your first morning, thankfully.

The child psychologist stops by just before lunch. She is an affable lady. She rings a bell in Evan's ear, but there is no obvious response.

'Ah well,' she says, gently, 'we'll try again another time', adding, 'You're his mom, you know him best, so we want to know what you see.'

What a lovely change of pace from the ICU.

Plenty more people, in various colours of uniform, come by throughout the day, and almost every one of them asks me if Evan is awake or napping. Each time I have to explain that no, he hasn't woken up in a month — I really wish they'd read the file first.

Then come the therapists, Occupational Therapy (OT) and Physical Therapy (PT). They work on Evan together, giving him a good stretch of various limbs. They tell me that my holding him is the best therapy he can get because he is calmer with me (as opposed to a stranger) and because it gives him a sense of where his own body is, as it curves against mine. It is the first time in a long time I have felt useful.

Later, Angela R from infant stimulation comes by to introduce herself. She has an extra sensitivity about her that is as surprising as it is unfamiliar among the professionals I have met. She tells me she will start taking Evan to school in a few days. 'School' is the playroom a few short steps from our room. It crosses my mind that a child's first day at school is an important moment. I wonder if I am ready for it. Then I remember where I am and why. I realise that 'firsts' for Evan will be different from the 'firsts' I had imagined when he was born.

Finally, we have a visit from the Speech Therapist. She introduces herself with a very husky voice: 'I'm Evan's speech therapist. I'm not sick, this is my voice.' She sticks foam lollipops in Evan's mouth, and pushes her gloved fingers down on his tongue. Although nothing in there is working, she says she thinks she could feel his tongue pushing back a little. Then she runs her fingers along his jawline on the outside and he moves a little.

Towards the end of the day, a neurological consultant comes by and examines Evan. He is a small, very slight man, in a pink shirt that seems one size too large. He tells me he has been to Scotland and enjoyed it very much. Do I have any questions for him about Evan? 'Not likely, mate,' I want to say, but instead I venture forth with, 'The lids of his eyes sit ever so slightly open. Do you think this means he is coming to?'

'Probably not,' is the swift, though not unsympathetic reply.

A nurse's assistant, Andrea, comes in close to 5pm with a large blue tub on a cart and announces it is time for Evan to have a bath. Andrea is Jamaican and in her late forties, with a warm and friendly nature. She tells me to watch how she bathes Evan as I will have to do it myself once I get settled in.

'Splishy splashy sploshy, give yourself a washy,' she sings out, uninhibited, as she manoeuvres Evan's wires and cables, covering him in soapy bubbles, before rinsing him off and taking him out to dry him.

21 March 2012

I go out for a walk today to try and get more of a feel of the area. You can't really call it a neighbourhood, it's so deep in suburbia that there aren't any pavements. The hospital is technically in Valhalla, but the 'main drag' of the town is about two miles down the road. There are two routes there. One takes you in between two graveyards (Jewish on the left, gentile on the right). The other is between the gentile graveyard and a school campus, although the school itself is set so far off the road that there is very little sign of life there either. The main drag boasts a train station, a couple of restaurants and a garage. Up here, beside the hospital, are two garages, a pizza place, a Chinese takeaway, a dry cleaners, a deli and a wooden restaurant called the Cabin. Manhattan it is not.

The hospital has a newly built wing, which we are in. It only opened four months ago. There are two babies to each room and the room itself is kind of 'L' shaped, with one half by the only window, looking out onto a fairly deep row of trees which, when their leaves come in, might just shield us from the view of the freeway beyond. The other half — our half — is by the door, and gets the majority of foot traffic. There is a large private bathroom to the side, in between the two halves.

Our room-mate is a small baby boy called David. He has some kind of gastronomic problem. I overheard someone say that it's like very bad acid reflux. He has a feeding tube through his nose. David screams through the night like he is on fire. His parents don't sleep over. There is something quite disorientating about being woken up by someone else's baby when your own is only ever silent.

There is also something odd about sleeping in a public place, as I have been doing for over a month now. My couch bed was originally right by the door, but today I pulled it round to the other side of Evan's bed, next to the bathroom. With the curtain around our section pulled over, we have more privacy than before. It is certainly better than sleeping on full display as I had to do in the ICU.

Still, there's no getting round the fact that you're sleeping in public. You have to wear suitable clothing, and you have to make sure you are safely covered by your bedsheets; you hope you don't snore, and you hope you don't talk in your sleep. None of the staff care whether you are sleeping or whether they are making too much noise. And, because the primary purpose of the hospital is to care for the sick children, and you are just a guest by the bedside, you really can't complain. So I don't. I also make a mental note not to feel bad about getting up past 10am.

22 March 2012

I spend today feeling sick about the ACS court appearance tomorrow. There was a time when I would look forward to a court appearance for days in advance; when I would spend hours preparing a case, sleep little the night before in healthy anticipation. I would show up at court and hopefully do something good for the client who, maybe, might come away happy. Now I am the client and it doesn't seem likely I will see happiness (courtroom or otherwise) any time soon.

Randi calls to say there is no way ACS will drop the case against me because they can't rule out the fact it might have been me who harmed Evan. She tells me they believe the odds are 50/50 as to whether it was Norma or me that shook him. This isn't anything different from what ACS had said to Randi at the first court date, but it still catches me off guard. Somewhere along the way I have allowed myself to believe this particular part of the nightmare might just end without further incident. But no, here it is, raging up against me once again.

I feel winded at the fierceness with which this has returned, and wounded all over again at the accusation. The thought that there can be any question I could have hurt my wee boy makes me feel physically sick. The fact that there doesn't seem to be any way to prove otherwise scares me. And despite all of this,

I just can't convince myself that the babysitter I knew, and had grown fond of, hurt Evan. That makes it all the more terrifying. If I can't, in good faith, point the finger at her, then of course the finger will be pointed at me. There was no one else involved.

How am I supposed to prove it wasn't me? I know from years of lawyering how hard it is to prove a negative. I can prove I wasn't with Evan after 8am on the day this happened, and we know the ambulance came between 4.30pm and 5.15pm, and that Norma had been with him in between.

According to Dr Brown, no one is sure of the onset time of SBS – from act to effect, how much time can pass. I was alone with Evan from 5pm the evening before. We had had a lovely time, but there weren't witnesses available for that. There was the nice young man who passed us by, outside the Lincoln Center on the Upper West Side, and said, 'That is so sweet', as he saw Evan and I gazing lovingly at each other. There was the lady in Gap, who Evan had smiled at. I had no idea who or where they were. And no one had been with Evan and me as we sat and laughed and cuddled on the couch later that night, opening up our brown paper package tied up with string. And anyhow, what would proving all of that do anyway? Absolutely nothing at all. My lawyer's logic has left me. And all the hurt and fear has consumed me once again.

Evan's social worker stops by our room and finds me crying.

'Bad things happen to good people, Elise,' she offers.

Later, Pauline phones me just to check in, but she can tell how bad things are.

'I know this is awful, Elise, but you don't have the luxury of falling apart right now. Evan needs you to be strong and you're going to need to get through court tomorrow. You can fall apart at some point further down the line, but you just can't do it right now.'

She suggests that I go and find a light bulb to change. Her point is that, when you feel everything is entirely out of control, doing a tiny thing like fixing something can help. I don't have a light bulb handy, and if I did, knowing my luck it would break. I'm very aware that I shouldn't be trusted with broken glass right now. I suppose the mental distraction of this train of thought pushes me past the darkness of the moment for long enough to dilute some of the despair I was in at the start of the call.

Liz, Jackie and Deborah all send kind and encouraging texts. Eventually I manage to pick myself up and gain some strength, not for me, but for all the friends and family who are rooting for Evan and me. After all the effort to help us, the very least they deserve is to see me keep going.

23 March 2012

Jackie has arranged to come up from Manhattan and drive me back down there for court today. She is such a star. She once told me (years ago) that a friend of hers had been running in the New York Marathon and she went along to cheer her on. At sixteen miles, the friend got into real difficulty and wasn't sure if she could run much further. Jackie jumped over the barrier and ran the final ten miles with her friend – in jeans and worn-down sneakers. That's our Jackie. She would do anything to help a friend in need.

As promised, she arrives at Blythedale this morning. She has a Manhattan coffee and a muffin for me. She drives me to downtown Manhattan, where all the courts are, and we meet Randi in a coffee shop twenty minutes or so before the hearing. I didn't sleep well last night and I am still anxious, but I have calmed down a little from yesterday. I feel very out of place, surrounded by lawyers with their suits and briefcases, all talking to their clients or on their phones.

Randi and I try to talk strategy. She thinks she can find an expert who could cast doubt on whether it is SBS or not. I tell her it seems like the wrong stance to take. I don't think there is much point in trying to challenge Dr Brown – she seems pretty sure that it is SBS, and so do the army of doctors who have treated Evan since. Besides, that will also take all the focus off Norma, and I want to know what happened when Evan was in her care.

When we go into the courthouse we have to wait in the lobby outside the courtroom as we have done before. The stress of the first experience comes flooding back and the conversations circulating around me begin to make me feel light-headed. 'Termination of parental rights', 'Custody of the State', 'Accept a finding against you and move on'. I don't feel strong enough to hear any of these words, but I know I have to keep it together. The last thing I can afford to do is get hysterical in front of ACS. They will only use it against me to say that I am highly emotional and therefore could have hurt

Evan. Instead I do the very unnatural thing and sit and listen to it all. I only scream inside.

Randi returns from a conversation with Lubin and Weaver. Nothing has changed since yesterday and they still have no interest in dropping the case against me. Neither of them can give a reason why they haven't brought a case against Norma yet, although, Randi reports, Lubin at least looks a bit embarrassed, in her opinion, that Norma is still gainfully employed as a babysitter, and still looking after other infants of Evan's age.

Randi reports that she reminded the two lawyers of my diligence in taking Evan to the doctor several times, but that Lubin had responded, 'That could be a case of Munchausen by Proxy.' In other words, it might have been a double bluff to disguise my hurting Evan, or as part of some attention-seeking stunt.

Everything in my world has been turned upside down.

She reports that Lubin mentioned that both Dr Brown and Detective Reyes have been less than communicative with him, and he doesn't know why. I would have thought that was pretty obvious. They have both made it clear to me that they were thoroughly annoyed at ACS having brought charges against me, especially the manner in which they had done it, dragging me down to court, away from Evan's bedside. How could Lubin not work that out for himself? He is young, he is inexperienced, I think. And then I remember the power he wields over me.

As we wait, Randi hands me a medical form, which I must sign in order to allow Columbia to share Evan's medical information with her. It is already prepared and lists the names of all the doctors she could think of. I read through them. I read the name 'Dr Grim'. Apparently Randi heard us talking about the neurologist at Columbia but didn't know 'Grim' was not her real name. The laugh that generates calms my nerves quite a bit.

The court officer comes into the lobby and calls, 'Parties on Schwarz!'

In the courtroom, I have to suffer the humiliation of identifying myself as the Respondent once again, but still feel my usual pride at adding that I am Evan's mother. The judge is, again, nice enough towards me, and, like last time, very short with ACS and Weaver. He seems genuinely concerned when he asks how Evan is doing. Nothing much happens in the courtroom, except that we set another date, in June, to come back, and do exactly this, all over again.

And then we leave.

There was a time when I knew that a scheduling conference is nothing to get excited about.

25 March 2012

Dr M stops by this afternoon to say that Evan's respiratory effort is very poor — all his breaths have to be assisted. This means that the vent has to pump pressure in and out in order to get him to breathe. She says she hopes that all the stimulation he is getting will bring back the breathing.

I feel weak. I miss Evan, I just desperately want my boy back.

26 March 2012

I hold Evan all day long, every day now. I felt quite self-conscious at first, because you have to make sure all the tubes and wires are in the right place and don't get disconnected. But once you get the hang of it, it's lovely. I sit in the visitor's seat next to his bed, propped up by pillows on either side. Evan sits in my arms and I pull the table over and rest a magazine on it and read. I talk to him as much as I can and, so long as it feels private enough, I might sing him a little song or two. I read somewhere that babies can hear and learn in their sleep, so there's no harm in trying to see if that applies when they're in a coma. I also read in that same article that they can breathe and swallow at the same time, too. I am trying to ignore that part, since Evan can do neither right now.

27 March 2012

In the ICU, Evan was entirely unresponsive to anything at all. He's been showing little improvements since he came to Blythedale. Today, every one of his fingers reacted to being squeezed. Speech Therapy says all his toes on the left foot are reacting and some on the right too.

This afternoon, Dr M transfers Evan to a portable vent. This means he can now travel to school and be with the other children. Between this and all the other tiny little improvements I cry tears of joy.

Later, I feel just optimistic enough to go online and do some research of my own. I try to find out why Evan's eyes won't move. Apart from that one time in the bath, there hasn't been any movement at all. It turns out that patients in comas should have an 'oculocephalic reflex'. That means that if you move their head one way the eyes will move in the opposite direction. It's also known as 'dolls' eyes', which is a good description. Anyway, Evan doesn't have it. If you move his head, his eyes stay exactly where they always are, dead centre. And here lies the danger of internet research for the under-qualified. I read that absence of the oculocephalic reflex in comatose patients is indicative of a very poor prognosis.

28 March 2012

Angela R came to get Evan ready for school today. It took a lot of preparation to get the portable vent ready to roll. All in all, it probably took a good fifteen minutes to get from Evan's room to the schoolroom, just ten yards away.

There can be between one and six babies in there at any time, some on vents, some not. The ones on vents have to sit near the wall because they get plugged in. Each child benefits from the stimulation of being part of a group, but gets some one-to-one time as well.

In school, Angela R tells me about her son, Saliman. He is eleven, and she has a daughter who is thirty-two. 'Angela is old,' she tells Evan, making a funny face. It turns out that Saliman was a baby in Blythedale and was born with his legs folded behind him. As a result, they had to be amputated through the knee.

He had other conditions too, and was facing years of surgery. Angela fell in love with him from the start and that was that. She adopted him and he's been the love of her life ever since. She tells me about how she treats him like any other kid, and ignores his disabilities. One time they were in the supermarket and he fell and landed smack on his knees. Because he landed on the prosthetic, it made a huge sound and everyone turned round to see if he was okay. 'Get up, Saliman,' she said. 'Everyone was looking at me like, how can you be so cruel?' she laughs. In fact, she was just treating her son as she would any other eleven-year-old horsing around in the supermarket.

If you saw Angela in the playroom you would know instantly what she brings. She doesn't take no for an answer. Evan is still in a coma and she has him rolling around, rattling toys in his face, singing to him, like he was any other baby. What makes her different from any other therapist in there is that she knows the pain of seeing your child less able than others, and the importance of giving them everything you can to make it better.

On the way back to our room Evan's eyelids open again, ever so slightly, but a little more than usual. Angela and I both say at the same time, 'We see those eyes!'

29 March 2012

Mini Perspective Day. Now we are here. Overall, not much has changed with Evan in the last ten days; a little tiny movement here and there. I realise that the benefit of having a perspective date is not so much to see how things end up looking on that day, but for the way it allows you to steel your emotions – even if just a little – until you get there.

I'm getting a bit more used to things, I suppose. I change Evan's tracheostomy ties tonight for the first time. It's quite a stressful process, but they have to be changed twice a day otherwise a fungus can build up on his neck. There is an outer tie that connects to the tracheostomy tube via two rubber strips at each end, which connect to two plastic buttons on either end of the tube about an inch away from Evan's neck. This is really simple to change. Then there is an inner tie that connects to the part of the tracheostomy closest to the hole in Evan's neck. You have to loop that through either side of the tube, right at the point where it sits on Evan's neck. This would be simple except while you do so, the tube itself isn't secured. So you have to hold it in place, in his neck, with one hand, while you change the ties with the other. If the tube slips out, Evan loses all breathing ability. You can try and push it back in, but it's floppy; the hole can contract and you might not be able to get it in. In that case, you have to reach for a new tube, which has a removable piece of hard plastic inside called an obturator or an inserter, which allows it to remain stiff while you insert it in the hole. If the hole really has contracted, then that tube will not go in and so you have to grab a smaller tube and hope you can get that in instead. While you do all of this, Evan is without any breaths at all. Therefore, as you might imagine, it is important not to let go of the tube when you are changing the inner tie.

Later, the eye doctor examines Evan. She says that his right eye has a haematoma in the middle, which, she explains, is not where you want it to be. It could block out all but his periphery vision in that eye. But, she adds, it is too soon to predict whether it will have a lasting effect. She says his corneas are fine and his left eye only has a small haematoma around the outside, so that's not much to worry about.

1 April 2012

Evan has a high fever today, at 103. He is writhing about. His tracheostomy is infected. You can even smell it. They raised his breathing rate to 30. His heart rate was at 191 at one point. I spend hours just wiping him down with a cold, wet cloth. His heart rate lowers a bit and then, with a few hours of cuddling, it comes down even further.

Once he is calmed I set myself off, thinking about how much I hate this situation. I want to be at home in our apartment, cuddling Evan on the couch, listening to his fat little chuckle, and watching his big blue eyes explore the world.

I am so tired of trying to be positive. I have begun to find it more and more difficult to be in a good mood for visitors. I am so sick of my natural inclination to try to make other people feel okay about this godawful situation.

And these anti-depressants – yes, they give me a cushion, but right now I just want a regular mood cycle. My son is brain damaged and pretty much non-responsive. I haven't heard him laugh or cry in more than six weeks. I need to be allowed to get into a very bad mood.

And so I do.

It comes on fast and strong. It is like the anger that has been so conspicuous by its absence in these last few months finally finds a way to burst through the anti-depressants and bubble up inside my psyche. I have reached my inner demons. They are pleased to see me.

I make a list.

1. The person I love with my entire heart is in a coma with brain damage and there is no guarantee of improvement.
2. Apparently, someone did this to him and the authorities seem to have forgotten about pursuing her.
3. I am charged with child abuse and I have no evidence in my defence.
4. I don't have custody of my own child.

And, of less significance.

1. I am slowly going crazy staying at the hospital every night.
2. I have lost my business – which I spent five years building.
3. I am about to liquidate every asset I have just to keep going.

Why did my beautiful boy have to suffer this horrendous damage? We were the happy ones; we didn't need to learn any lesson. I didn't need to appreciate Evan more. I appreciated every second of our short life together.

Anne calls. I offload on her. She is very good at listening. She makes lots of sympathetic noises and doesn't try to reason with me or to get me to see the bright side. There is a time and a place for that too, but not at this point in time. I need to feel my anger.

2 April 2012

I wake up feeling overwhelmed with guilt for getting angry last night. It feels like I let Evan down by not staying 100 per cent positive for him.

I never feel angry when I am holding Evan. As a matter of fact, that's the time when things feel at their best. When we are together we are not victims. We are love. We are strength.

4 April 2012

Evan is over his fever, so I decide to go back to the apartment for a break. I haven't been there since the day a grenade was thrown into the centre of our lives.

Jackie and Deborah come and collect me and drive me home. Jacques, the apartment building's doorman, meets me at the entrance and, without saying anything, gives me a huge hug. I manage to hold it together, just about.

I go into our apartment, alone, and sit on the bed, next to Evan's crib. I can hear myself sobbing loudly, long before I can feel myself doing it.

'I will bring you home,' I keep repeating, through the salty tears.

After a long time I settle down on the couch to take a nap. I don't wake up for 14 hours.

5 April 2012

The apartment building manager is letting me move to a larger apartment – a one-bedroom – two floors up. (When I say 'letting me' I mean, of course, that I have to pay a vastly increased rent and add some to my security deposit too, but it is a lot easier than it would usually be to find a new place in Manhattan.)

I speak to a couple of maintenance guys about the move. They have already been interviewed by ACS and by the NYPD, and know just about everything that anyone else knows.

Mike, the super, comes to visit and ask how Evan is. He's been in the apartment several times when Norma has been there, sometimes when I haven't.

'What did you think of Norma?' I ask him.

'I only knew her as a kind, very loving person,' he says.

Well, that had been my take too.

As I leave the building to return to Westchester, I bump into another maintenance guy in the lobby, also called Mike. He had seen Evan being taken out in the ambulance. His eyes fill with tears as I try to explain how Evan is doing. So do mine. Eventually I tell him everything will be fine. That cheers him up.

I return to Evan, delighted to see him, and feel refreshed and almost normal. As soon as I lift him up, I notice his eyes move – they move in the opposition direction to the way I move him. The doll's eyes have finally arrived! I am ecstatic. The 'poor prognosis' of their absence has gone, I think.

I call for Dr M, and when she arrives (with SW in tow) I show her the evidence of Evan's newfound oculocephalic reflex. She holds Evan and looks at his eyes. Then she puts him down in his bed.

'Let's go into the private family room and talk,' she says.

When we get there the three of us sit down.

'The eyes,' she says, not catching mine, 'I don't think that's a good thing. I think it's a sign that the eyes and the cortex are not talking to each other. That he can't see.'

I am shocked. I had read that this can be an implication of the oculocephalic reflex too, but come on, surely we can at least celebrate getting to here, and we can worry about neurological blindness at a later stage. As usual, though, my emotions overwhelm me. At least this time I know better than to try and argue the point in the state I am now in.

But that isn't the end of the conversation.

Dr M continues, 'Unfortunately, we don't think Evan is improving fast enough.'

'What?' I manage, 'but he's doing so much!'

'Yes, well, you see, he's not doing enough. He needs to have voluntary movements and we haven't seen any yet.'

I try to protest, but there really isn't anything to come at her with. Evan is improving at glacial speed. In the ICU, when I first saw him make tiny movements, I thought we were at one out of ten. Then I thought we were at one out of a hundred. Now it's clear we are moving in increments of one thousandths – when we move at all.

6 April 2012

One of my best friends from Scotland, Angela B, arrives with her husband, Neil B, today for a visit. It is lovely to see them, but the emotions of the moment as well as the lingering effects of yesterday's conversation with Dr M are too much and I burst into tears before I can even say hello.

Once I calm down we go for lunch and I fill them in on just about everything – except the court case. That just feels too much of a distraction from Evan.

Or, more honestly, I feel shame around it.

Later, back at Evan's bedside, Angela B, trying to be positive, asks me, 'What is his best thing?'

'Nothing, Angela, he has no best thing right now. Look, there's a chance that this is as good as it gets.'

I think my frankness shocks her a little. It shocks me a bit too. I feel any confidence I have managed to muster in these last few weeks has taken a big knock since yesterday's conversation with Dr M.

7 April 2012

I am so weepy this afternoon that I have to text a visitor, Gail, and tell her that if she hasn't left home yet, not to come. But she has just arrived at Valhalla train station, armed with a big bag of fruit. 'Look,' she says, warmly and kindly, 'how about I drop the fruit, say hi, and then leave again?' She does, and it is a comforting visit. She only stays for twenty minutes and knows to leave me to it. Sometimes it amazes me how sensitive and kind people can be.

8 April 2012

EASTER SUNDAY

Angela B, Neil B and I walk across the highway to the Cabin for Easter Sunday lunch. As soon as we sit down, I see a baby at the table across from us and I break down mid-sentence. Angela makes me change seats with her so I won't have to keep looking at the baby. I am in tears, and so is Angela. The waiter comes over and Neil B asks him to just give us a minute please. Neil B is crying too. 'It's all just shit,' I say. 'Nothing will ever be good again.'

We manage to right the ship eventually and the chat turns to Celtic Football Club, of which the three of us are huge fans. Football has filled the unforgiving minute for us more than once before.

11 April 2012

I come back to my apartment for a break from hospital life, hoping Angela B and Neil B might be there. Neil B has already said they won't: 'No, you need your own bed and I couldn't stand it if we had your bed and you slept on the couch. No.'

Neil B is possibly the most thoughtful person in the world, not just for that, but for so many things he has said and done along the years.

I sleep deeply through the night and wake at a whopping 12.54pm. When I eventually get myself up and out, I go to an unfamiliar coffee shop. I can't face going to my regular one in case the girl behind the counter asks me, 'How's the baby?' as she always used to do.

It is beginning to feel quite a mixed bag, coming home. I need sleep. I need the break. But I miss Evan so very much. I know I need to rejuvenate myself. If I can't get to a more positive place in myself, I can't help him. I miss him all the time. I have to keep reminding myself that I have not lost him.

12 April 2012

I get back to the hospital and hold Evan. His little head is moving ever so slightly. I can feel it against mine. It is almost like he is nuzzling in. SW comes in and I show her. Again, I find that there is something not quite connecting about her. Then Angela B and Neil B and Angela B's sister Martine come in and Angela B notices that Evan's fingers are very loose. We all sit and watch them for a bit and then, blow me, the fourth and fifth fingers on his left hand actually move – and keep moving.

What a high! We even catch it on video. Neil B gets so excited you can actually hear him say the 'f' word during it – who can blame him?

Dr M is in the room already, being harangued by the parents

of Evan's room-mate over nothing in particular. I am very patient, despite my huge excitement, and wait until she finally comes over which, because she has to pass us to get out of the room, is a given. 'Look,' I tell her, and, graciously, Evan does it again. She laughs kind of nervously and then says, reluctantly, 'Okay, I'll put it in the book.'

As she turns to leave she stops and, pointing to me, tells my guests, 'This is a woman of great hope and conviction.'

'I hope I'm not alone in that,' I reply.

She leaves without answering.

13 April 2012

Evan is making lots of noises from his mouth today. Since his mouth, jaw and tongue can't move, it's only his voice box that's producing them. They call it 'phonating'. I film it. Later, I put his plastic splits on his hands, and his face becomes blotchy. At the same time, his heart rate shoots up to 124 (from about 90). I feel awful – his splints must be annoying him – but at least he is able to communicate this. I take his splints off and get him out of his crib for a cuddle. He relaxes in my arms and starts to look much better.

I start thinking that Evan and me are too alike in this scenario. He lies in bed and is really no trouble at all to the nurses – very low maintenance – unlike his room-mate, who gets a huge amount of attention from the nurses because he screams so loudly and painfully. I am low-maintenance, too. I never call the doctor in, I never complain. Our room-mate's parents call the doctor in every single time they come to visit. I am not a squeaky wheel: I need to be.

So, when most of today passes without any therapists coming in, I decide to make an issue of it. At 4.45pm, when PT comes by, I tell her it isn't good enough that no other therapists have shown up all day. She, of course, isn't one of the culprits, but she looks very sorry anyway. This makes me feel bad for the rest of the evening. Still, it's a start. I have to get used to putting Evan's needs above anyone else's.

14 April 2012

Saturday night: Angela B and Neil B's last night. I come back to the city and Neil B graciously lets me sleep on the couch on this occasion (I really do insist). Liz and Deborah join us all for dinner at a nice wine bar close by. As I sit there at the head of the table, facing into the street, with nice open windows, hearing the laughter and chat all around me, I feel an almost overpowering urge to take my wine glass and throw it as hard as I can so that it smashes on the pavement outside.

16 April 2012

I feel resentful of Dr M right now. It feels like she holds all the cards when it comes to Evan's improvements, and yet she walks past his bed every day to see David, without stopping to see us. And I hate the way she answers all of my questions beginning with 'Mnnyeah…' It's like she is reluctant to say the word 'yes' in case it sounds positive. I alternate between three avenues of conduct I could take with her. I could trust her and assume they are working on his vent settings, and that they are doing things behind the scenes that I don't understand. Or I could blast her like a hair dryer and start demanding real changes (although I have no idea what they might be). My third choice is to be passive-aggressive and just sit and stew until one day I blow a fuse and accuse her of doing nothing for all this time. Ultimately, for now, I end up doing nothing anyway, because my depression sneaks in and confuses my thought process and I literally lose the plot.

To top off another bad day, my cover gets blown at the Cabin tonight. I've been going there a lot. It's the one part of the day when I can pretend all of this is not happening to me.

Tonight, the waitress, Trish, who I've been chatting with occasionally, asks, 'So do you live around here?'

'Kind of,' I reply.

Then I give her the brief version of how and why.

'Is he going to be okay?' she asks.

God, how I hate that question.

'Yes, I hope so.'

She is very sympathetic and concerned. Nonetheless, my anonymity is gone. I can no longer pretend I am someone else when I go there. I might as well walk in with a banner above my head that says, 'Sadness and Pain'.

Blythedale

18 April 2012

I wake at noon today in my apartment. I had to come home yesterday – I felt exhaustion getting the better of me again. The first thing I do when I wake up is to call the hospital. I've come to realise what an anxiety-inducing procedure that is.

Me: 'Hi, this is Evan's mom calling to see how he is.'

Nurse: 'Hi, how are you?'

Me: 'Fine, thanks, how are you?'

Nurse: 'I'm good, thanks. Are you at home?'

Me: 'Yes, how is Evan?'

Nurse: 'I'm not actually Evan's nurse today but let me get her for you…'

Another nurse: 'Hello, yes, this is Evan's nurse, how are you…'

…And on it goes until ten to twenty seconds of my life have passed with my heart in my mouth.

Eventually, today's nurse says Evan is having a good day.

I sign the lease for the new apartment and then go for breakfast at the diner round the corner on Amsterdam. They are showing a football game on their TV screens and I am watching, starting to relax and enjoy it. Then I see one of the players stick out his lower lip in a show of dissatisfaction at a call. It reminds me of how Evan used to do that if he didn't like something, and I have to leave.

I go back to the apartment with a coffee and sit on the couch. There are two books on my bookcase that raise an ironic smile when I think of them. One is *What to Expect: The First Year*, which is a guide through the first twelve months of a child's life. It has thoroughly missed its mark as far as Evan and I are concerned. The other book is *What To Do When Things Fall Apart*, which, if you ask me, is an understatement of my life as I have come to know it.

I stop looking at these books and instead look down at the lowest shelf. Something is sticking out from the space on the ground beneath it. I reach down and pull out a plastic baby-sized oxygen mask and tube. The paramedics must have left them behind. Next, in a scrunched-up ball, I pull out the pyjamas that Evan had been wearing the last time I saw him smile. They have been cut off him.

20 April 2012

This has been going on for nine weeks. When will it stop?

I get back to the hospital and Evan is in school. I go and watch him from the windows that wrap around the room. He looks as comatose as ever. It hits me very hard this time, even though I see him like that all the time. It actually shocks me.

Later, when Angela R has finished her exercises with him, I take him back to our room and hold him tight. PT comes in and I know I will break if I have to have a conversation, so I leave her with Evan and I walk over to one of the graveyards. I get about a mile in and sit by a little pond.

Days like this — days without faith — leave me feeling desolate. Hope is better. The effort to remain positive is usually worth it. But there are days, like today, when it feels like there is nothing to hang onto, no strength left. The darkness creeps over me and I can't remember what it feels like to live in light.

As I sit by the pond I start to wonder if God actually wants me in heaven. Would he really give this kind of pain to someone he expected to remain on earth? I know I have very little will to live any more.

By the time I get back to the hospital it is dark and the night shift have come on. I feel absolutely twisted with grief by this time. Evan is just the same as when I left him, but I know I can't pick him up. I am scared that if I do, I will infect him with my negative energy.

Instead, I lie on my bed in the dark. The demons quickly come to get me. They are much stronger than the devils; they attack from within.

I can't lose them. It feels almost as if they are trying to burst out of my skin. Eventually I reach into my closet next to the bed and pull out a pair of scissors. They are the only sharp things I have. I draw the blunt blade across the inside of my left forearm. It feels painful and strangely cooling. I take the blade and press down as I run it across my ribs. That is sorer, but it doesn't feel sore enough. I don't actually draw blood. I have a couple of red welts, that's all. If I had something sharper, I would have made a better job of it.

As I lie back on my bed and let the pain soak in I think briefly about why I have just tried to harm myself. I know there is a theory behind why people cut themselves. I know it's got something to do with getting the pain from the inside to show on the outside, or that it feels good to heal in some way, if you can't heal in the way you want to. But when I drew those scissors on my skin it didn't feel like any of that. It felt like the emotions I was experiencing were so strong – and so awful – that there weren't any words to describe them. If there had been, I would do what I always do when I'm upset, and write the right words down. No, there are no words, only a painful act of expression.

Somehow I fall asleep. I dream I am in the front passenger seat of the ambulance again, racing up the West Side Highway, with Evan in the back. The only difference is I am not in shock this time, as I had been then. I can feel everything. I can feel the fear as raw as it is possible to feel anything.

I wake up, to an almost eerie calm. It's like I have come through some kind of feverish delirium and am now well rested. Although, more than that, it is as though I have come through a level of hell but have made it to the other side. The demons are gone.

21 April 2012

I have therapy today. I've been going for a few weeks. I have applied for disability benefits since I can't work, and so I have to go to therapy to show that I am truly depressed. I don't mind, it's a good place to decompress. My therapist, Debra, is tall, very slim and has well-chosen clothes. She has a nice house, a beautiful golden retriever, and a Honda in the drive with a Democratic sticker on the bumper. It's easy to imagine that she has the perfect life (I think most therapy patients believe that of their therapists at some point in treatment). She is warm and caring, and I'm always worried she may have taken on too much when she met me.

I've been to therapy before. I spent three years of my life sitting on a couch in a therapist's office just south of Union Square. We had muscular sessions where things were worked out, shallow thoughts exposed, and entire ways of thinking abandoned and replaced by something healthier. But these therapy sessions are nothing like those. Now I go in and cry and dump my problems of the week on the floor and Debra takes out her broom and sweeps them into tidy piles for me.

Today's session is good. I tell Debra how low I felt two nights ago. I don't tell her about the scissors, but I feel a lot better anyway so there isn't any need. She reminds me that when you get depressed it's not possible to see that things can get better. Unless Evan gets better, I don't think things ever will be, not really.

23 April 2012

SW pays me a visit and asks for permission to speak with Evan's Legal Aid attorney about my case. 'Evan has only one advocate, and that's me,' I tell her, more in rhetoric than in realism. I sign the document anyway. What choice do I have? This sets me off on a course of apprehension about the upcoming court compliance conference. I have come to terms with the fact that nothing happens at these appearances. What I now dread, though, is having to read the Blythedale letter prepared for the court and all parties, updating Evan's medical status. There is never anything good in it.

At least the day ends well. My massage therapist friend Rebecca visits and gives Evan a massage. He is visibly more relaxed than most nights and is soft and cosy when I take him in my arms. He is out of it – yes, of course he always is – but this feels different, more sleepy than comatose-y.

25 April 2012

I take another break in the city, and sit in a local bar watching the second leg of the football match I had watched part of last week. I am feeling nicely distracted by the screen and a refreshing beer when I receive an email from Randi. She tells me ACS has amended the petition. She doesn't know in what way. She tells me she will get back to me.

I feel so entirely helpless, and actually terrified. I want to leave the bar, but I feel too scared to even stand up. I worry that ACS has decided to try to terminate my parental rights (Randi had told me that it was a remote possibility). I try to keep reminding myself I didn't do anything wrong, but the threat of losing Evan is just too big to be able to rationalise.

An hour passes before Randi emails again. She tells me the amendment is to add the babysitter to the petition, and bring the same charges against her. The relief is overwhelming. When it feels that my legs might work again, I get up and leave the bar. I go back to my apartment. I still have no idea what the final score was.

Blythedale

27 April 2012

Jackie drives Deborah and me to court. We meet Randi in the coffee shop again and she is surprisingly, and refreshingly, positive. She is delighted that charges have been brought against the babysitter and feels it can only help me.

As we are talking, I show her some recent photographs of Evan on my phone. She looks and then pushes the phone away, padding at the make-up on her eyes with a napkin. 'I can't cry before court,' she says. It looks like it might be a little too late.

I am more relaxed today than I have been at past court appearances. For the first time in this process, something appears to be happening that favours me. As we sit in the hallway, waiting for the case to be called, I feel relaxed enough to take a look around. I see a teenage boy emerge from a courtroom with what looks like his mother and his lawyer. The boy has a black eye, and the mother looks as though she has been crying. The lawyer draws them over to one side to continue his conversation with them. Another attorney comes into view. She has a shaved head, a short skirt and a short-sleeved jacket. Her legs and most of her arms are bare but covered in colourful tattoos. Many of the attorneys look quite poorly dressed compared to the attorneys in the courthouses I am used to. Amid all of this, Randi stands out in her stylish black clothes, and her sparkling diamond jewellery.

The court officer steps into the hallway and calls, 'Parties on Schwarz!' (Norma has not yet been served and so is not required to attend today). We follow the officer back into the courtroom. The judge starts the proceedings as soon as we sit down. The Weaver lawyer – 'Evan's lawyer' – shows up late, and spends the entire time giggling into her file (I don't know at what). To top it off she plays with her hair in what is, to me, the most annoying fashion.

Randi stands and asks the judge for a protective order against the babysitter. Now that she has been served with the petition she knows where we are, and Randi doesn't want there to be any risk of her visiting us at Blythedale. In the past I would have said Norma isn't the type of person to do that. These days, I know nothing for sure and I don't stop Randi.

The judge turns to Weaver and asks her if she has anything to add. She manages to get herself entirely on the wrong side of the request for a protective order to aid her client (Evan) by stating she doesn't see the need. Then she smooths her blonde hair some more. The judge rolls his eyes and grants Randi's motion anyway.

He directs the lawyers to get their calendars out so he can set the next compliance conference date. As is typical in a courtroom with three lawyers and a judge, it takes some time to find a date on which all four are available. The judge is very accommodating when Randi and ACS say they have conflicts on certain dates, but when Weaver announces she is unavailable, the judge rolls his eyes again and says, impatiently, 'Just get someone else from your office to show up.' This is a fair point. She has added nothing to the proceedings to date.

Court is eventually adjourned and everyone prepares to leave. 'Legally Blonde' Weaver walks past Randi and me and I can't resist taking a pop at her: 'If you think you represent my son you are doing a very shoddy job.'

This apparently shocks her a little and she replies, 'Well, like, I feel bad, but I don't know what's going on in this case, like…'

Well, of course I just about have a fit at this.

'You have done nothing for my son,' I say, my voice stronger now. I can feel myself close to losing control. The judge intervenes, and tells 'Legally Blonde' to go out into the hallway. He turns to Randi and says, 'Ms Karmel, you will control your client.'

I calm down a little and manage to say, 'Judge, I'm very sorry, I just feel very emotional in this situation.'

'Perfectly understandable,' he says, with more than a hint of sympathy.

As I head towards the door, he adds, 'I completely understand.'

It feels good, though, to let some of my frustration out into the court's cold air. It is actually quite exhilarating. Weaver, of course, is not really the source of all that built-up anger, but she certainly does a very good job of turning herself into a temporary target.

We walk out of the courtroom and into the street. Randi hails a yellow cab, we hug; she jumps into it and disappears. Jackie, Deborah, Liz and I walk back to the parking lot amid the many lawyers, in their suits, with their trial cases and their associates, all coming from or going to one of the several other courthouses in the area. I begin to yearn for all of that again: the excitement, the suits, the preparation, the walk up the courthouse steps. The feeling, on leaving, that you just did a great job.

I get back to Evan and feel refreshed — as though I have had a brain shower. It feels so good to hold him, and to know I am bringing some really strong positive energy to him for a change. His fingers and hands are all moving, as is his right foot. As usual, the movements are tiny, but it adds to my exuberance. I feel strong — like I really can cope with all of this.

'Ehhh-vaaaan, I see your momma's glad to see you,' I hear Andrea singing out from the doorway as she watches us cuddling. I tell her all about the day. She finds it very entertaining.

30 April 2012

Last night, as I was lying in bed, the nurse started arranging Evan's toys in his crib. She was doing it with great enthusiasm, to the extent that the bed was shaking. I couldn't stand it after a while and leapt up and told her to be gentler. She was quite surprised to see me pop up from the other side of his crib like that. 'It's okay, he's my baby,' she said, in broken English. 'No, he's my baby only,' I told her, almost hissing.

In retrospect I'm sure I was over-reacting, since she really wasn't doing him any harm. I lay back down and watched her Crocs passing by at the bottom of the dividing curtain. She was actually tip-toeing. I felt awful. Then I started sobbing, hard, but trying to keep silent. I had finally come to the realisation, after months of denial, that Evan had been hurt by someone and that I hadn't been there to protect him. I cried deep into the night.

Even though it doesn't feel like it, I suppose I must have slept a bit because I did manage to have one of my awful dreams about

Evan. I can't remember all of the details, but these days I mostly dream that he dies.

Anne arrived from England this morning to stay for a week and to allow me to go home to Scotland to see our mum for a few days. I have been really looking forward to her coming, even though I am only going to get to spend a little bit of time with her before I leave.

I wake up to find her already sitting at the other side of Evan's crib. I shower and we go out to get coffee. We get a couple of steps outside the hospital doors and she bursts into tears. She hasn't bargained on being so shocked to see Evan in this state again. And, fair enough, although I have become relatively used to it, Evan hasn't really changed much since he was in the ICU. His face still doesn't move at all, the dolls'-eyes thing is actually quite creepy looking, and most of the time his eyelids still sit two-thirds shut. Nothing else moves much either. I think my occasional videos of him make it seem like he has improved a lot more than the reality.

I can see the pain on Anne's face. As usual, I start crying too. It turns out that we both just need a good flush of tears, because after that we are fine, relatively speaking.

We get our coffee and bring it back to Evan's room. We are met there by the bright and cheery Dr M and SW in advance of a 'family meeting' that was planned some time ago. They invite us back to the small windowless room with the round table and chairs, and this time all four are put to use.

I have been thinking about this meeting for a few days, and had planned to get in the first comments and try to direct the conversation. But, having just finished crying with Anne, I have lost concentration.

Dr M manages to get the first word in.

'Unfortunately...' she begins, quite ominously, 'Evan had issues at the weekend where he desatted a lot and at one point, worryingly, his heart-rate plummeted.'

This is true, and I was there.

'Perhaps that's because the nurse forgot to take off his old medicinal patch when she put on a new one and the extra dosage is what led to the drop in his heart rate.' (Also true.)

'Oh, mnyeah,' says Dr M, having obviously overlooked this. 'That was unfortunate.'

This is possibly my 'in' to assert myself in the conversation, but she is too good for me, and continues on without missing another beat.

'Evan is not making the improvements we hoped he would make.'

Oh, here we go again. Naturally I try to argue but she keeps going.

'As a result we are reducing his therapies down to three sessions per week per therapy.'

'You have got to be kidding!' I am incensed. 'If you don't see a change then keep doing it until you do.'

'It doesn't work that way,' she says.

'Then don't give him any therapies at all,' I counter.

'It doesn't work that way either,' she says.

I change tack and cut to the chase. 'Is there anything I can do to make you change your mind?'

'No,' she replies.

'Then this meeting is over,' and I storm out of the room with Anne following close behind.

At the door I stop, turning back to Dr M, and say, 'Evan and I are on a journey to his recovery – you're welcome to come if you want, but we're going there anyway.'

Once I get back to the safety of our room my bravado subsides and the emotions come flooding back. As I sit holding Evan, and crying, Angela R comes in. She is comforting and consoling.

'I still have hope,' I manage to say.

'Your hope's your hope – you keep ahold of that – nobody can take that from you,' she says, hugging Evan and me together.

1 May 2012

We have to go to SW's office this afternoon to sign a Power of Attorney giving Anne the right to act in my stead while I am in Scotland. Once we sign it, SW suddenly hands me a 'Consent to Refer' form, approving Evan's referral to one of two long-term care facilities (one nearby in Yonkers, the other in Wanaque, New Jersey).

'If it's "consent" that's needed then I don't consent,' I tell her.

'Well, if you won't consent we will have to get ACS involved,' she responds caustically.

Shocked, I try to gather my thoughts. I don't want ACS involved in decisions about my own child.

'I want to speak to my lawyer first. I'm sure it can wait until I get back from Scotland.'

'Does ACS know you are going to Scotland?'

She is playing her trump card. She knows I am desperate for this break to see my mum and she is issuing nothing less than a thinly veiled threat that she can somehow jeopardise it if I don't do what she wants me to do.

'Don't talk yourself into a bad position here,' I warn her, to no effect.

She delivers the stinger: 'If it wasn't for the ACS hold, you could take him home now.'

This is said as a taunt. SW's face is sneering. There is no response to it, so I walk out of this meeting too.

I go back to the room. Anne draws the curtain around us and I weep and weep. Angela R comes in and sees me sobbing for the second day in a row.

'They're kicking us out,' I manage to say. 'But we can't go home, they're making Evan go to a long-term care facility.'

She can see I am broken at this. She knows as well as I do that a long-term care facility is a step down for Evan. There will be fewer therapies on offer. There is no bed for a parent to stay the night. Whether she knows it or not, I am convinced that if Evan goes to one of those places he will never leave. Angela R walks out and two minutes later in walks the supervising nurse, again, presumably at Angela's request.

The supervising nurse draws the curtain for privacy and explains to us that, although the hospital might think they are done with us, the reality is that Evan is still on a vent, and there are no vent beds available in any of New York's long-term care facilities right now, so it might be a while until it actually becomes a reality. This makes me feel a whole lot better.

2 May 2012

Realising any move will not be imminent, and also that I really do not want ACS to be involved, I have a brainwave this morning and call in Dr M. When she arrives, I go over all the things I feel are lacking here at Blythedale (mostly to do with the reductions in Evan's therapies), none of which she can argue with. And then I tell her that, as we're getting no love here, we might as well check out, so yes, I'll sign her form and we'll take our chances elsewhere.

This allows me to save some face before signing the consent form.

Dr M looks uncomfortable at the confrontation. I am not uncomfortable with it at all; I am furious at the lack of belief I've felt from her. It is good to realise that the crippling fear that kept me from talking to any doctor at all back in the ICU has now gone. I'm a little better armed with knowledge than I was before.

Later, after the form is signed, I wheel Evan into school, where he gives me a big treat by moving his eyes to the side, twice (properly, not dolls'-eyes style). I leave him there and then go back twice to give him extra kisses. Then Anne walks me to the front door and we have a good hug.

At the airport, as I sit waiting to board and trying not to freak out, I call Anne. She has been holding Evan non-stop since I left.

I Believe in Evan

8 May 2012

I'm almost at the end of my trip home. It's been so lovely to see Mum. She was still in bed when I arrived, and Mary, her daily carer, came in and saw us hugging and filled up with tears.

Mum and I sat on her bed, catching up on how the journey had gone, and how Evan is doing. After a while she pointed down at the floor to her side, at a handful of books that were wedged between the side table and the wall. 'See those books? I dropped them down there the day you called to tell me Evan was sick. They've lain there ever since.' I picked them up for her.

Margaret, Mum's cleaning lady for the last twenty-five years (and an adopted family member) arrived a few hours later. I went out to the hall, where I found Mary and Margaret talking in hushed tones, about how I was doing. When they saw me, they both looked like they'd been caught with their hands in the cookie jar. I was very touched by the conspiracy.

People came to visit me at Mum's over the next few days. Some asked directly how Evan was. Others waited for me to talk about him. All were very sensitive and very caring, and all treated me quite delicately, which I needed and appreciated.

As comforting as this trip is, sadness stays with me the entire time, some days hanging heavier than others. My bedroom at my mum's house has Evan's cot in it and all the toys I had left behind for the visit we'd planned ten weeks ago. There are some clothes here, for age six to nine months, which he should be wearing now, and some books I should have already been reading to him but haven't.

Still, I really needed this break. I needed to be with my mum, gentle and kind and funny. Usually, when I come home, we have a day or two of struggle as I try to persuade her to go out for lunch. I always win, but we both get a little bruised in the process. (Emotionally, not literally. God, ACS would have a field day with that one!) This time, though, I have had no desire to go out into the world, and Mum has been quite relieved at this.

Instead, I have been happy to stay indoors and wait for Anne's calls and texts. I have had at least five conversations with her each day, several by Skype, where I can see Evan too. Anne knows to launch into a report about Evan on pick-up, so I don't have to wait and worry while we get the formalities out of the way.

9 May 2012

I am back with Evan, and it's wonderful. I've been telling him story after story, letting him know about everyone who was asking after him. He seems quite a bit more alert than when I left him.

'Ehhh-vaaaan, I see you getting kisses from your momma,' Andrea sings from our doorway. I am pleased to see her too.

Randi emails, saying she has contacted ACS to see if there is anything they can do to prevent Evan going into long-term care. They have already replied that no, they won't get involved. They don't mind taking a child away from a loving innocent mother, but no, they draw the line at trying to make things better. (Okay, they didn't say that last bit.)

10 May 2012

Evan is very drowsy today, after having been so alert yesterday. They've started giving him Ativan because he has been arching his back a lot and they are concerned it might be some kind of seizure activity. The Ativan makes him ridiculously droopy, and I'm very wary of over-medicating him. I speak to Dr M about holding off on the Ativan. She tells me it's up to me. I still don't quite get this doctor/parent relationship. I can tell them what to do about things I don't know anything about – medication – but the common sense stuff (don't reduce his therapies, he needs all the movement he can get) are apparently beyond my authority. Ultimately she proposes we stop the Ativan and to give him an EEG. I am not entirely sure how this transpires but I agree.

11 May 2012

We have been moved to a better room, more space, further from the door and all the foot traffic it brings. I have a feeling the supervising nurse did this to help me feel more secure about our tenure here. Our new beds are at the window, and we now get natural light. This is an amazing concept if you've been sitting in the dark end of a room for close to a couple of months, as we have. Also, our new room-mate is a very premature (and therefore tiny) baby girl. The only sounds I hear from her side of the room are the occasional coo or soft cry. It's a million times easier to share a room with her than with poor wee David the wailer.

Blythedale

The only issue with this new room is that my bed is now in full view of the hallway, where there is constant foot traffic. People stare in as they walk by. At night I have to remember to pull the curtain right around Evan's bed so I can sleep with some privacy. That's not always possible. Whenever there is an issue that is too serious to handle without help, the nurse (or me, if there is no nurse) hits a blue button next to Evan's bed. This is dramatically known as calling a 'code blue', or a 'rapid response'. At Blythedale, as soon as the alarm sounds, everyone (doctors, nurses, technicians and sometimes even secretaries) comes rushing into the room. Sometimes you can hear the alarm in other rooms and then you wait and see people running up and down the halls. Even when I know my child is safe I experience strong anxiety at the thought that another child is in danger. When the code is over, I always ask if everything is okay. The nurses know they are not supposed to divulge any information about another patient, but the kinder ones always give me a little nod to reassure me.

In the middle of last night Evan's nurse had found herself in the wrong position when changing Evan's trach and had to sound the alarm. Before I knew it there were sixteen people in the room. At least my decision to wear a bra to bed during this whole period has been vindicated.

I Believe in Evan

13 May 2012

MY FIRST MOTHER'S DAY

Dear Evan, in a few years we will go over the rules of Mother's Day, but for now it's enough that I can hold you in my arms and kiss your gorgeous soft skin.

At Blythedale I don't get the steady flow of visitors I did at the ICU. Company was crucial for me then, but here's more of a space for quiet reflection. I ignore a lot of emails, phone calls and texts these days. I always used to wonder about people in crises – why they didn't reply to my heartfelt messages to them. I'd imagine they were consumed by things to do and just didn't have time. But it's not that – I do nothing but hold Evan all day long.

I suppose I just don't have the energy to engage with most other people. Instead I rely on people's goodwill and the fact that I seem to have a lot of licence right now, and I do nothing at all. A bigger reason, though, is that, as the weeks have rolled on, I feel more and more dismayed by what people aren't saying rather than what they are saying. Gradually the praise for Evan's tiny movements has disappeared. It is replaced by praise for his clothes, or for the layout of Blythedale. I can't stand it.

Every now and then I do get a visit, though. An old friend from San Francisco, Edel, popped in a few days ago. She lived in the same apartment building as Gerry, Violet and myself. She is in Manhattan on honeymoon and made the trip up to

Westchester to see us. As with any of that group of friends, the years fall away every time we meet. I didn't feel the need to soft-soap the situation for her, and the two of us just spoke naturally. It was a relief not to have to put a brave face on, which I realise I almost always at least try to do.

Jackie and Deborah visit every few weeks and occasionally manage to persuade me to go out for dinner with them. Rebecca still comes and gives Evan a massage as often as she can and if I'm not in a foul mood I'll go for something to eat with her as she waits for her train back to Manhattan. Liz comes up once a week from Brooklyn and often catches me in a good enough mood to go out for a drink, although I usually make her listen to me rant. My friend Brian lives nearby. He knows a lot about sport and can distract me quite well with a beer and a decent game on a television in a nearby bar.

I suppose what all of these people have in common is that they understand our situation deeply. They ask nothing of me, and often they get very little in return. But it is comforting to know that they are there.

14 May 2012

Evan's breaths per minute have been dropped to twenty-eight, and his oxygen rate has been reduced too as he seems to be satting well. These are good changes.

Speech Therapy reports having had a good session with him today, and that she got some kind of response almost every time she touched him. She tells me this with not inconsiderable delight. She has been eating a Jolly Rancher sweet and her tongue is the colour of her blue eyes.

Evan's eyes open more often now, for a few minutes each time. They still don't actually move much on their own, but the fact that he can open and close them now is something. He attends school today, after speech therapy. When he returns his eyes are almost fully shut and his heart rate is very low. He is exhausted.

I've become very tired of my evening walk to the Cabin for dinner. For one thing, you have to walk through Blythedale's grounds to get there. Twice a night I pass by the same rusting memorial, partially hidden in the bushes. It appears to be some kind of swing ball set, although it's clearly been broken for many years. It has a plaque on it, saying it is dedicated to some poor forgotten child who died in 1974. Its dilapidation is even more depressing than the various memorials throughout the hospital (on pieces of medical equipment usually), which memorialise other little dead children. In this kind of setting, no parent needs these constant reminders of the very worst-case scenario.

For a change of scene, I've started walking all the way down to the main part of Valhalla and back each night. I stop for a couple of beers in the bar down there. It's a four-mile round trip and I probably balance the calories in with the calories out. It takes care of several hours each evening and gives me something to look forward to.

On the way there I walk down the road that separates the two graveyards. It's still daylight at that time. On the way home, when it is dark, I walk up the other road, with the non-Jewish graveyard on my right and the school campus on my left. I never see anyone else walking, and there are no streetlights, but this road at least has a few passing cars to light my way every now and then.

Walking home in the dark from Valhalla is something I would never have done when things were normal. As a matter of fact, I used to do long bike rides, up to a hundred miles a day, and this stretch of country road, being so quiet, would have freaked me out a little bit if I was riding it alone, even in daylight. Yet here I am, a frequent traveller of it now, alone, in the dark, with a graveyard to my right. On the very best nights the moon throws some shadows on to the road through the tall trees and bushes that shade me from the north end of the graveyard. There are never any people around. Sometimes I feel like I'm daring the universe to send a bogeyman to come and get me. Only the threat to Evan scares me now.

15 May 2012

In therapy today I was talking about how things cannot be awful forever. Whether Evan gets better or stays like this, we have to reach a comfort level, surely. I can get used to this, if this is what I have to get used to. But as I don't know what it is I have to get used to, I can't get myself to that sense of settling. The uncertainty is terrifying in itself.

I don't actually mind if Evan is disabled – I love him enough to deal with that. But I can't see him as anything less than perfect and I wish the doctors would see him as I see him. What is their view of perfection worth anyway, or anybody else's view? I'm certainly not perfect and I don't know anyone who is. Don't we all use only about twenty per cent of our brains anyway? Who says a boy on a ventilator can't bring you as much joy as a boy on a bicycle?

And why is Dr M so negative all the time? Why can't she say something like, 'Look, I don't think he is going to improve, but I think you can adjust and in time the two of you can reach a stage where you can both be happy'? Next time she wants to 'chat' I'm going to give her a blue Jolly Rancher first and then I'll just focus on the blue on her tongue instead of listening to her doom and gloom. Maybe I can get Andrea to put on a white coat and stethoscope and tell me exactly what I want to hear: 'Everything is going to be just fine. And by the way, Evan is the most beautiful baby in this hospital, by far.'

20 May 2012

I moved most of our things from our home into the new apartment a few nights ago. I was surprised at how good it felt to do something so physical. I loved living in that little studio apartment, and it was a perfect apartment in many ways, tiny though it was. I spent my happiest times there, because my happiest times were being pregnant and then, better still, being there with Evan when he was well. But I'm not sad to be leaving it – I don't want to remain in the apartment where this happened to Evan.

The new apartment isn't all that nice. It's dark (it's on the internal side of the building) and just doesn't have the same nice feel to it as the last one did. I know it's going to be months until this new apartment is filled with Evan. In the meantime it isn't home: it is nothing without him.

I get back to Blythedale, aware that the results of Evan's EEG should be in. I have dared to dream of good news. I am hardly through the door when Dr M comes trotting in. The first few words out of her mouth include 'unfortunately' (as always) and 'abnormal'.

Apparently Evan's EEG doesn't show much more activity that it did in the ICU. I feel flattened. 'Okay, thanks,' I say, and wait for her to leave. Then I sit alone with Evan in my arms and tears rolling down my cheeks.

Jackie and Deborah arrive to take me to dinner in Tarrytown. I tell them about the EEG, trying not to cry at the same time. Jackie can spin anything. 'Well, isn't that better right now than if he was having a lot of activity but couldn't express it?'

Good point, Ms Frank.

21 May 2012

Evan is still as fully ventilated as ever, but he no longer needs to have oxygen added to the flow. I don't exactly understand this, other than that it's a step in the right direction. Sometimes he gets very red around the eyes. I think he might be crying, but because his face doesn't move and his eyes can't even blink, this is as much as he can show.

I have been giving people some prayer cards that my sister

in Scotland has made for Evan. His smiling face is on the front, with a prayer to St Anthony. There's a little prayer on the back too. It's nice to have something to hand to people when they ask about Evan. In a way it gives me a brief break from explaining everything.

We have a new nurse, Madison. She never smiles, but she seems to find great joy in pulling my curtain open in the morning so everyone out in the hallway can see me sleeping. She is good with Evan, but I am fast learning that she is unencumbered by compassion for parents.

23 May 2012

I had to go home to the apartment this morning. I have a cold and feel sick and achy and dizzy. They are very strict at the hospital – if you are sick, you have to leave because there are too many vulnerable babies around.

This afternoon I call to check on Evan and on whether anyone had reduced his 'breaths per minute' rate. I'm hoping that now that he doesn't need extra oxygen, if they lower the rate of the vent he will start breathing on his own. I've been trying to pin the doctors down to start reducing his settings. I know nothing will get done if I'm not there to bug them, so I'm dedicated to making a real pain of myself by calling in as much as I can. True enough, when I call this afternoon, they haven't reduced the rate at all. So I leave a long message with the nurse practitioner. I call later and they have decreased the rate to 20 breaths per minute.

25 May 2012

I am still sick. And I am hating being away from Evan.

I have had this apartment for a week now and notice tonight for the first time that it doesn't have a microwave. As the kitchen is six feet long and two feet wide, I'm surprised I ever thought it might have one.

As I'm holed up in this soulless apartment while I try to get better, I've been trying to work through the bags of clothes transported in the move. I've been wearing the same few clothes at Blythedale for a couple of months now, and should change them now I have the opportunity, but I can't be bothered.

Since this happened to Evan, my standards have clearly been slipping as far as my appearance is concerned. I used to spend hundreds of dollars a month on my hair, getting it cut and coloured. I spent more on clothes, though – mostly for work. I also used to do some form of exercise at least three times a week, usually swimming, cycling, running or a combination of at least two out of the three.

Now I find myself wearing clothes I wouldn't have been seen dead in before, like baggy flannel shirts, old and unflattering T-shirts. Last night I went to meet Liz but it was raining. I put on a fishing-style hat a friend had brought back from Africa and walked all the way to Times Square in it. I attracted many looks from the fashion-conscious but didn't care. It was very comfortable and it kept the rain out.

Dress sense aside, I have certainly looked better physically. I know I wear my pain on my face, but I also suffer from lack of sleep at the hospital. When I took a cab to Valhalla train station the other day and the driver asked me if I lived nearby, I replied, 'Long story but no, not really.'

'That's a pity,' he said. 'You look like you need to go home and sleep.'

Other than my evening walks (motivated by the numbing beer in the middle) exercise doesn't ever cross my mind. I am physically immobilised by sadness almost all the time.

With nothing to do in the apartment I've been looking in the mirror a lot. Earlier today I stood for a long time, gazing at my misshapen outline, my puffy face, my untidy hair. I have at least an inch of white roots showing. So that's how it happens, I thought. How people go from youthful to middle-aged and do nothing about it – because it comes to them in the midst of having to cope with something more important. I really just don't care how I look any more.

23 May 2012

Another day at the apartment due to illness; I am beyond upset. My emotions are so raw, I cry constantly. But it doesn't help: I just want Evan.

I've spent most of today getting wound up with thoughts of Blythedale. I need to go back and tell them to focus on Evan more. I need to demand that the vent be taken to task.

29 May 2012

I finally feel well again and am back at Blythedale.

When I arrive, I rush in to see my baby boy, but Madison is with him and, quite typically, takes her sweet time with him before handing him over to me. Once I have him in my arms, and have hugged and hugged and hugged him, I called Madison back in and asked her to get Dr M for me. Madison takes great delight in telling me Dr M is on vacation. 'Is nobody covering for her?' I ask through thin lips. She calls the replacement doctor, who comes right away, and listens to my concerns about the vent. I tell her everything I have spent the last few days thinking about. I add that I am tired of us being ignored. I tell her I need action by Friday or I will file a written complaint.

She gets right on to it all immediately. She spends about an hour with me as she works her way through the file and says professionally artistic things like, 'It could be a little bit of perspective, but I hear you loud and clear.' She eventually works out what the issue is, and it isn't one I have prepared myself for.

No one really thinks Evan can ever get off this vent and that's why no one's trying.

30 May 2012

I am still licking my wounds from the vent conversation yesterday when the rehab doctor comes to see me this morning. I met him on Evan's first day here and haven't seen him since. After introducing himself (he has obviously forgotten that we have met before) he tells me, in as many sentences as he possibly can, that no, he won't increase Evan's therapies because he doesn't see any improvement.

'Well, since you reduced his therapies by two-fifths, don't you think there might be some kind of correlation with his lack of improvement? I'm not the one in the white coat, but I do know that if I put forty per cent less gas in my car than normal then I can't expect it to go all that far.'

This is my best analogy, but it doesn't win the war we are waging. Dr Rehab comes back with seven, eight, maybe nine (or even ten) more sentences, all spoken in monotone. Eventually he says, 'I have no authority to increase his therapies.'

As New Yorkers would say, that was a long way for a shortcut.

'Then can you please send in someone who does have authority,' I ask.

'I don't send people in,' he says, in a tone that reveals his increasing annoyance at the conversation.

'Then ask the person who sent you in to send in the person with authority.'

Okay, clearly this conversation has degenerated and I am not going to get anything on my terms. That reality notwithstanding, Dr Rehab isn't going to leave on anyone's terms but his own and sits for another ten sentences or so until I am not only dejected but also thoroughly bored.

Still, a few months ago a doctor telling me there was 'not much improvement' would have, and frequently did, leave me in tears for hours. I came to the refreshing realisation after my conversation with the immovable Dr Rehab that my skin is a lot thicker now. As well as being a lot more haggard looking.

Another doctor, Dr J, pays me a visit later in the afternoon. She is a friend of a friend and works in admin at Blythedale, but is a neurologist by trade. I think she must have heard about my visit from the doctor yesterday, and about my conversation with Dr Rehab today. I whine a bit (she has a sympathetic air about her). I can't touch the vent issue, though – I have no counter-attack for that at all – and I can't take all the bad news that comes with a conversation about it.

I tell her I'm really annoyed that the therapies have been reduced. She is very candid. She tells me that no one knows whether therapies work at this stage. When someone comes in with a brain injury they treat it aggressively and give as many therapies as possible. But if they see there isn't much change they reduce them. She says it could be that the brain is not yet ready to heal in those ways. Also, it might not be such a good thing to stimulate him as much if he isn't quite ready for it.

We talk about long-term care and my concerns that it would feel like giving up on Evan. She says she doesn't see it that way, that it could be that Evan just needs more time to heal and can do it best there. I still don't buy that. I tell her I don't believe Evan will ever get out of long-term care if I allow him to go into it. She says if they start to see a significant improvement as a result of the therapies, they will keep him here.

I ask her about the dolls-eyes' issue. Is it good or bad? She says that it's good if you are in a coma because it shows the brain stem is working, but if you are not in a coma and you have it then it means the eyes are not connecting with the cortex. I ask her if she thinks Evan is still in a coma, and she says she isn't sure, that there are various degrees, and it is sometimes hard to tell. But, she says, 'We have time here.' She explains that the infant's brain keeps developing until they are two or three and whatever is going on right now, there's still time to correct it. She also says that it is a positive sign that Evan has dolls' eyes after not having any eye movement at all.

What a good feeling to have a conversation with a doctor that is not entirely negative. Even the parts that aren't totally positive still weren't like the 'chats' with Dr M (doom, gloom, gloom, doom). I wish all of Evan's doctors were like Dr J – although she isn't actually Evan's doctor at all.

31 May 2012

Evan's eyes seem to be more open and fixing a little. He doesn't always move them like dolls' eyes now, which is a good progression. Hopefully it means his brain is starting to connect with them more and more. I touched his cheekbones today and he reacted by moving his left shoulder. He particularly reacts to any touching near his eyes. His left leg seems to be doing something too.

Evan's ventilator alarm starts beeping as he lies in my arms. I look down at him. He has turned blue. I yell and the nurse sees it and presses the code blue button. I put Evan into his crib and step back. The room swarms with doctors and nurses. They bring him back round very quickly. 'He's pinking up,' I keep hearing them say. After the fuss is over they discuss what happened. They aren't entirely sure, but after looking in his nappy there is a common consensus that an over exertion in the bathroom department is the prime suspect.

I am inconsolable despite the humour. After five minutes attending to Evan, the on-call doctor and several nurses sit with me for about twenty.

Once I have calmed down a little I am able to sit and hold Evan again. As I grip him tight, SW walks in. She tries to make conversation with me (as though there was no bad blood at all), but I can't speak, not even to tell her where to go.

5 June 2012

I visit Elizabeth Seton Pediatric Center. Yesterday, when they called to confirm my appointment they also confirmed that, no, they don't have a vent bed available for Evan right now. I actually did a little dance. So now, safe in the knowledge that Evan can't be sent here until they have a bed for him, I feel quite relaxed.

It really is a spectacular place. The rooms are spacious and bright. There are therapy rooms for everything. It even has a large whirlpool room with a hoist to lower children into it from their wheelchairs. I imagine how soothing the water must feel on their bodies, and how their limbs are free to move to just the gentlest of resistance in there.

As impressive as the facility is, though, the visit doesn't change my mind. Evan and I need to take our chances at getting out of Blythedale and getting home. Another hospital is not the answer.

I head back to Manhattan after the visit, but I call to check on Evan first. Madison tells me he has had a desat – just to the early eighties, and is fine. He has had a couple of these recently, but no one seems too concerned. I guess desatting is just part of life on a vent.

7 June 2012

I've had another few days back in the apartment. I feel rested and ready to come back to Blythedale this morning. I take the train to Dobbs Ferry and start a long sun-filled walk over to my therapist's house in Ardsley for our session. The plan is to head to the hospital once we are done.

My phone rings when I am halfway there. Dr M's cheery voice says 'Hi' on the other end.

She is on speakerphone. SW is with her.

'Is Evan okay?' I ask before I say hello.

'Yes, yes, he's fine,' is the friendly, relaxed response. 'We're just touching base with you.' She explains that she has just returned from vacation and has heard about Evan's several desats recently.

'Mnnyeah, it appears his brain is shutting down.'

I am, needless to say, floored by this.

'What? Can't there be another reason?'

'No, he's not looking too good. I don't see any of those breaths he sometimes takes. It's not a good prognosis for Evan.'

None of this, incidentally, is said in anything other than a matter-of-fact kind of a way.

'Wait a minute,' I manage. 'What about the fact he's been weaned off oxygen? Or that we've been reducing his BPM over the last few weeks – even if it's by just a bit, it's still all in the right direction.'

'Mnnyeah, we'll talk when you get back, then.'

'But you called me – out of the blue. You will stay on the phone and talk through this.'

'Mnnyeah, well…'

I can tell she isn't going to give me much more. I don't think she really thought about the consequences of her call when she first made it. Still, it is hard to know whether I have her against a wall or she still has me against one. Instead of ending the call there and then though, she changes tack and asks, 'Do we have a DNR for Evan?'

This is a 'Do Not Resuscitate order'. It would prevent any lifesaving measures being administered to Evan in the event that he suffered another cardiac arrest or other life-threatening episode. There is no way that Dr M does not know whether there is one or not (there is not).

'Do you see a DNR in Evan's file?' I ask, sharply.

'No, I don't.'

'Because there isn't one, and that can't change without me, right?'

'That's correct.' Her tone is more subdued now.

'I'll be back in an hour.'

Even though I don't fully believe her, the thought of losing Evan is just too much. I get myself to therapy and start crying right away. Poor Debra. She has to wait for me to explain what just happened. When I do, she is shocked.

'They told you that over the phone? But you're always there!' I keep crying.

'Don't forget,' she says, 'They've been wrong before.'

Well, that is a very good point, and it calms me a little.

After an hour of trying to thrash out what the phone call is all about, we end. I leave with my head a little clearer, but still very upset. I don't want to take this upset to anyone else – it seems too much to put on friends and family, after everything else they have had to witness. I feel so alone.

I get back to the hospital and pick Evan up from his crib. As far as I can see, he is every bit as good as when I left on Sunday. His cheeks are rosy, he is taking the same amount of occasional breaths that he has been doing for a while now, and his vent settings are exactly the same as when I saw him last. He is also reacting well to my touch. I go out to the hallways to fill my water glass. I meet Dr M and SW as they happen to be coming out of Dr M's office.

'How are ya?' SW sings out cheerfully, if entirely misguided.

I ignore her and turn to Dr M and say, 'That should never have been a phone conversation – I think you are wrong, but regardless, you should never have delivered that news on the phone. I could have been anywhere.'

She at least looks cowed, and quite considerably so.

'I just wanted to touch base, it's been a long time since we talked.'

I don't give her an inch, though. 'I am here all the time. That should never have been a phone call.' And I walk away, knowing that I am right.

8 June 2012

Dr M makes a point of coming to see us this morning. She still looks cowed. I go over everything with her, about how Evan no longer needs added oxygen; I still see him take the occasional breath; his colour is usually good these days; he doesn't desat anywhere near what he used to.

'I just don't know what it is you think has changed?' I ask her when I'm done.

'It was just a perception,' she says.

This is actually fairly decent of her to concede. I have experienced plenty of doctors who wouldn't concede anything at all (Dr Grim and Dr Evil, for two). Even though she falls far short of what I want her to say, which is, 'You're right, I'm wrong', I do not slam her. God knows, I could, but I know I still need her onside for Evan's sake.

Finally, though, I have a little firepower.

'There are no beds for Evan at Elizabeth Seton, so Evan and I are in here for the duration. You and I don't have to agree, and Evan doesn't have to perform any tricks to stay here any more, but it would be very helpful if you could give us some positivity while we are here,' I tell her.

Later, the nurse practitioner comes in. 'I hear he went blue again and that he's desatting more and more these days.'

'No, dear, you're a day late and a dollar short.'

I do have to confess though, that when I left four days ago for my break, I was slipping into a little bit of complacency. I was contemplating spending more and more time at the apartment.

This, I guess, is a wake-up call – Evan needs me here, even if it is just to protect him from the negativity of the doctors.

There is a certain release in knowing that it no longer matters what Dr M thinks about Evan now. He can't be shipped off to Elizabeth Seton as there are no vent beds. He can't be sent home because of the ACS action. (I find it hard to imagine that any doctor would be so irresponsible as to discharge him right now, given that there are still some very frightening episodes, but apparently the medical insurance company thinks he would be just fine.) Foster care might be seen as an alternative to him coming home with me (and I can imagine few things worse), but, because there are no foster carers in New York who are proficient in using ventilators, that is not an option. He is stuck here at Blythedale, where he is safe, and where I can stay by his bedside for as long as he needs me. So the remand and the vent both actually help us.

The irony is not lost on me.

9 June 2012

He feels like the Evan I know, soft and gentle of spirit. Right now, Evan can…

1. *Move his left leg about a half an inch*
2. *React when you touch each cheek*
3. *Move his tongue – just at the very tip – it's really more a flicker than a movement*
4. *Fix his eyes*

5. Squeeze my fingers

... sometimes.

But he is beautiful all the time. And I never stop loving him.

Jackie visits and brings some fantastic clothes for Evan — lots of checked pants and golf-style shirts. He dresses up well. Black is a very good colour on him on account of his light brown hair, blue eyes and dark eyelashes. He has the palest skin. Evan has everything about me that I like, but he has replaced what I don't like about me with much better things. He has long legs. I have short, stubby ones. He has long fingers. Again, mine are short and stubby. He has well-proportioned feet. This is starting to depress me a bit. He has the same nose as me, but my nose has a freckle on one side, which I have always hated. His is entirely blemish-free and very, very kissable.

11 June 2012

Did a day's work today, on my last case. My client is smart, and has hired co-counsel for me. There is no denying that I am still not operating with a full deck these days. My focus is shot and my thoughts are always with Evan, no matter how many documents I try and read. Anyway, it's nice to know there's someone there to do all the legwork for me, so I can be with Evan as much as possible.

I travel all the way to Queens (about two hours door-to-door) for the hour-long meeting with the client and my new colleague. It goes fine, until I get an email from Randi: she has been in court on my case. It was Norma's first appearance, but I didn't need to be there. I had asked Randi to pass on a message to her: 'If she admits it, I will forgive her.' Randi's email includes Norma's attorney's response to my message: 'There is nothing to admit, there is nothing to forgive, she has excellent references.'

I need to stop believing the thoughts in my own head. Why did I think that Norma would own up to whatever it was she did just because I said I wouldn't be angry? Still, maybe it will plant a seed and make it easier for her if she does ever decide to say what happened.

I'm floored, though. There seems to something around every corner these days, waiting to give me a good swipe. Just when I think I'm doing a little better, I either get a call from the hospital or a communication from Randi about the ACS case. And I realise just how very fragile I am.

I pop an Ativan. It's the only way I can see myself getting all the way back to Blythedale without a major incident like a panic attack. I have such horrendous anxiety for the two-hour journey anyway that I shudder to think what would have happened if I hadn't taken the pill.

I am pleasantly surprised when I arrive. Today's nurse tells me that Evan has had a great day, but that she noticed recently he gets troubled by the secretions at the back of his mouth – if they don't get suctioned often enough, he can get a bit panicky when he tries to take his own breaths and that's why he has been desatting more than usual recently. She has already relayed all of this to Dr M, and has recommended a water flush after each feed.

Vindication.

12 June 2012

ACS called me today, to arrange a home visit. They have a new caseworker on. There was nothing to it really, but the phone call got me down anyway.

I have been thinking long and hard about moving back to Scotland with Evan when this is over. I want to feel safe, but I don't, right now. It's more than that, though. There is something just so deeply hurtful about being accused of hurting Evan. I don't want to leave New York just because of hurt feelings – I love living here – but perhaps we should take a break for a bit.

When it's all over.

13 June 2012

When I'm not sitting holding Evan (although I usually am) I have several routines here that help me get through the day. Sometimes I spend my evenings eating alone at the back of the hospital at a picnic table, out by the skips and the construction debris of the hospital's new wing. I buy a can of beer from the garage and sit in the dying sun, counting the fireflies.

When I have the energy to be in the company of others I walk down to Valhalla for some decent food. When I'm done I see how many complimentary mints I can grab as I leave the restaurant. Then I set off walking the dark road home. By the time I get back to Blythedale the mints are always gone. I hold Evan for another hour, and then we both go to bed – 'Up the wooden hill,' I tell him. Connie Connolly used to say that to me as she sent me off upstairs to bed for the night. Evan has only ever lived in an apartment or a hospital, so it wouldn't make any sense to him even if he could understand.

Another routine I have come to enjoy is my daily breakfast outing. Every morning I go to the deli and get a bagel. I used to then go to the garage and get a coffee. One time the bagel guy saw me in the garage and got offended because the deli serves coffee, too.

That's not what made me switch to bagel guy's coffee, though. One day I went in to the garage and the friendly guy who is always behind the counter, and who knows I live in Blythedale, asked me what my husband does. 'I don't have a husband,' I told him, patiently. 'What? What? But you have a baby, right?' To add to this, I was on the phone with my mother and had just put my phone on the counter to reach for some change, and she heard the entire thing. I haven't shopped there since (but I'm sure I will if I need something there I can't get anywhere else).

14 June 2012

I have finally had it with SW. I get back from therapy this afternoon to be told that ACS has been and gone. I know that they like to make drop-in visits where they don't announce they are coming, but this was not one of them. The nurse tells me the

ACS caseworker told her she had set it up with SW in advance. I call the Head of Social Work and leave a long polite message about how I would like a new social worker, please. I say I will explain in detail if required, but the long and the short of it is that I need someone new. Within an hour a tall blonde woman walks in.

'Hi, I'm your new social worker – can we start with a clean slate?'

'Well, not till I've offloaded onto you a bit first,' I tell her, revving my engine.

16 June 2012

Evan is teething! He has one tiny wee white ridge poking along his lower gum. I am so proud! It explains his agitation lately. Poor thing, he can't put his hands in there or get at it with his tongue. His eyes have been reddening a lot. It's a real shame that he can't just scream out. He sweats from his head too, and his hair gets wet. So we have all decided that when his heart rate is high, his face is red and his head is sweaty, it's time for painkillers.

Dear Dark Spot on Evan's top gum, right of centre,
I see you and I know you are harbouring a very sharp piece of enamel. We all have to survive, we all have a right to exist. But let me tell you now, if your enamel hurts my son, I will hunt it down and, however long it takes, I will smother it with a pillow and trade it in for cash. Be warned.

I Believe in Evan

17 June 2012

When I started taking anti-depressants the constant flow of tears stopped, although the sadness didn't. The pills usually make things more manageable. I'm not sure why, but right now the tears are flowing almost as much as they were in the beginning. One thing I can't stand about crying is that when I do it, I tend to hold my forehead or my jaw in my hand. Evan and I look very alike, and whenever I do that it feels like it's Evan's face I am feeling – it's the same bone structure – and it's like I can feel him crying. It's his agony that I am touching. I can't stand it. And then I cry more.

19 June 2012

I haven't been back to the apartment since Dr M's 'awful and inappropriate phone call', but for the last few days I've felt myself starting to unravel a little. I have a hearing day today – on my client's case – so I come back to the apartment. I am thoroughly miserable, though. Then, this morning, I wake up from a dream in which I lost my breadbox and realised I would spend an eternity looking for it.

After a coffee and a bagel I walk from 71st Street to 32nd Street in the bright sunshine. It isn't yet too hot. NYC summer mornings can be quite special before the heat overwhelms. The smell of fresh soap and deodorant is still in the air and no one has worked up a layer of grime yet. My hearing is in the conference room of an office near Macy's department store in

Herald Square. Everyone else walking to work looks busy and like their lives are fairly normal. I am walking towards the end of my career. And I am very far from Evan.

I guess litigating skills become innate. I haven't prepared much for today's hearing at all, but all the facts of the case come back to me when I need them to. It actually feels uplifting. My new co-counsel sits next to me, which turns out to be a lot better than I thought it would be. In normal times I would consider that kind of help a massive dent to my ego. But these are not normal times, and in fact it's the only ethical way to proceed.

I get back to the apartment in time to wait for ACS to turn up and conduct their 'home visit'. When they arrive, Ms Dominique (who I know from the early days at the ICU in Manhattan) doesn't make any eye contact. Pamela Turner ('Call me "Ms Turner"') is the new caseworker and she's as brash and bold as she can be. She walks in and immediately focuses on Evan's prayer card, which just happens to be on the coffee table. She lingers on it to the extent that something has to be said.

'That's Evan's card,' I offer, helpfully.

'But he's alive, right?' asks Ms Turner. This stings like lemon juice on an open wound. I look at Ms Dominique, who has the good grace to look embarrassed.

'That's very harsh,' I manage to say.

Ms Turner doesn't apologise, but instead she explains that one time she walked into a mother's house unaware that her daughter had died, and started asking questions as though she were still alive. She only realised her mistake when the mother handed her the daughter's urn of ashes. This does not make me feel any better.

They sit themselves down and Ms Turner says, 'So what happened in your case?'

Ms Dominique and I look at her.

'You don't know the case?' I ask.

'I do, but I want to hear it in your words,' she says. (I resist rolling my eyes skywards, but it is not easy.)

'Well, I got a babysitter, I went out to work, Evan had a cardiac arrest and was rushed to hospital, and when I got there I was told the babysitter shook him. All the doctors I spoke to said it had to have been the babysitter because of the time of onset, but ACS brought this case against me. The police don't believe it was me, and the investigative doctor doesn't believe it was me, but there you have it.'

After a few more questions, Ms Turner softens and says, 'Oh, this isn't a typical case at all. This isn't going to be too hard. We just have to get you and Evan back together again.'

Ms Dominique explains to her that I stay by Evan's bedside full time, but that there is a legal remand in existence. Ms Turner looks a little incredulous. 'Sounds even easier,' she says.

Ms Dominique tells her that Evan could be released home right now if it wasn't for the remand.

'Can you get a doctor to give a second opinion – that there's another cause?' Ms Turner asks.

I already know that this is 'possible'. Yes, I'm sure I could pay an expert to give a different point of view but I also know it is highly unlikely that this route will succeed. No doctor who has examined Evan has given me an alternative opinion, and an external expert could potentially write a report, but then would have a mountain to climb in court to combat all the opinions of all the doctors who essentially believe that there is no alternative. I tell Ms Turner this.

We revert back to talking about Norma.

'Well, she won't ever look after kids again,' Ms Dominique offers. This sounds almost like a claim to ACS success.

'Well, she's looking after them right now,' I remind her.

'Yes, that's true,' she admits, looking at her shoes.

'Well, look,' says Ms Turner, 'I will give my report to the lawyers and hopefully they will just agree to drop it. Then the judge decides what to do.'

This is all good news – especially as I have always felt that the judge is very sympathetic towards me.

20 June 2012

I get word today that I have been approved for monthly disability payments on the grounds of depression and anxiety. This is a big relief. I've been scraping by and the debts have been piling up. It won't cover everything, but it'll keep the wolves from the door for a while anyway.

22 June 2012

I have been doing some research online and came across a *New York Times* article about a couple of cases of SBS. One of the cases reported was about a boy called Noah, in Virginia. He was a victim of SBS-type injuries as an infant, a couple of years ago. His babysitter, at the time of the article, had been convicted and sentenced to twenty years in prison. She was waiting on the outcome of an appeal. Her lawyers had argued there was a reasonable question mark over whether she had shaken him (she maintains she didn't, and anyway, she was only with the baby for one hour in advance of the cardiac arrest) and, perhaps, whether it was even SBS. More searching led me to a blog called Noah's Road. It is written by Noah's mother. Noah is now three years old, and, apparently, has really very little wrong with him any more, although he did have some developmental delays.

What strikes me most about this blog, other than the fact that this boy is doing so well (which, of course, gives me great hope), is the fact that the parents are so incredibly angry. Maybe it's just the way the blog is written, but they seem to be only focused on the things Noah has difficulty with, and the fact that their younger son, for a while anyway, overtook him developmentally. Even now, a couple of years later, they are full of contempt for their babysitter. And she's serving twenty years.

My overriding emotion having read all of this is how grateful I am that I don't often feel anger. Hardly ever, actually, and only ever at what ACS are doing to me. I never feel angry about what has happened to Evan (immeasurably sad, yes, but not angry). With that said, I am aware I might just be living in a false dawn. Unless, or until, Norma starts talking, I really can't be sure what happened to Evan. I can say I can forgive her right now, and, right now, I believe I do. But, depending on what the truth really is, I may be being a little naïve. Perhaps her silence saves my sanity. There is also, of course, the future. What is it going to bring? How can I know whether this forgiveness that I am so certain of is going to stick around?

25 June 2012

I get back to my apartment and pick up my mail, which has been accumulating. I find a lovely card and letter written jointly by the mother of a friend of Pauline's and a priest, both in Glasgow. I have never met either of them. The priest writes that he used to play football with my uncle, back in the day, and that he will say a mass for Evan. These little things feel like stepping stones to me.

26 June 2012

I have a full day of hearings today, and again enjoy it, until of course I see a missed call from the hospital. I don't think twice about interrupting the proceedings to step out and return the call. Madison picks up,

'Blythedale Children's Hospital, Pod F?'

'It's Evan's mom – is he alright?'

'Hi, how are you?'

'Is he alright?'

'No. I mean, yes. They just wanted to increase his blood pressure medication.'

If this wasn't such good news inasmuch as it certainly isn't much worse news, I could jump down the phone and throttle her. I go back into the hearing, smiling, trying to assuage what are quite alarmed-looking faces.

28 June 2012

After a day back at the hospital yesterday I had to return to the city today for the third of four hearing days. Everyone involved – my client, the arbitrator and opposing counsel – have allowed the schedule to be spaced out as much as possible so that I don't have to spend more than one full day away from Evan. This case has been going on for years now, and is actually the most contentious case I have been involved in. Some of the attacks by lawyers (myself included) have broached the personal, which really shouldn't happen. I have no doubt that we have all hated each other on a very basic level at various times throughout. But, in this situation with Evan, I have to acknowledge the professionalism and kindness of all involved.

The hearing goes well, and, as I walk home in the heat of NYC, enjoying being part of the bustle again, I start to feel short of breath. I wonder if I am having some kind of panic attack. It comes and then it goes a little and I get myself home. When I get back in to my apartment though, I feel it again – like a constriction in my lungs – I can't really catch a breath. I stretch my back over the roll arm of my leather couch, trying to open my lungs up as much as possible. Eventually it goes away and I forget about it.

An hour or so later I get a call from the hospital.

'Is he alright?' I ask in my usual frantic tone.

A young male doctor speaks. 'Yes, he is now, but I'm calling to let you know he had to have a rapid response earlier this evening. He stopped breathing, even on the vent, and went blue. He desatted and his heart rate dropped to the low teens. We ambued him and he came back up. He's doing fine now.'

'Should I come back tonight?'

'There's really no need – he's very comfortable now.'

I ask the doctor what time it happened at. It was at exactly the same time I was stretching for air on my couch.

I take an Ativan and try to get to sleep, so I can leave as early as possible tomorrow morning to get back to my blue-eyed boy.

29 June 2012

I wake up feeling dizzy and not at all well rested, despite the passage of hours. When I get to the hospital, Evan is indeed fine and just as I'd left him. There's no hint of the drama he'd been at the centre of last night. I speak to the nurse who was on duty when the desat happened.

'The doctor wasn't going to call you but I told him he really had to. I told him you are a really hands-on mom and that you are always here. You're not like so many moms that don't want to get involved,' she tells me. Naturally, I thank her for being vigilant.

Speech Therapy meets me in the hallway later. She knows about the desat. She tells me that when she was working with Evan yesterday morning she had thought he was having a bad day – that she wasn't getting her usual responses from him.

I sit holding Evan, wondering whether to give in and let doubt overwhelm me.

Dr J pays us a visit, and we have a long chat. She explains that her view is that this is really a wake-up call to remind us that Evan is at risk of sudden death.

'That's not what we are focused on,' she continues. 'We are only interested in his rehab, but we all need to be aware that it's a possibility.'

There is something so genuine and warm about Dr J's manner that I can listen to all of this and still stay calm. She explains to me that Evan's brain is making new connections all the time, but some of them might not be helpful. She tells me that it could be that he is entering a phase right now in which he needs a little extra help.

Dr J has been the only doctor to date (other than my own therapists and Dr Brown, all of whom were supportive from the start) who has acknowledged how difficult this is for me. 'You've been through a lot,' she says. She tells me that she stopped giving prognoses in these cases a long time ago. 'It's not helpful, and there are always exceptions,' she explains. She adds that she does think Evan will have 'challenges'.

'Challenges' I can cope with. I've never shied away from a challenge in my life. It's lack of belief that's the killer. Dr J's manner is such that I don't divine an obvious dearth of it in her. That's what allows me to listen to her.

29 June 2012

I'm supposed to go to Glasgow next week. I booked it in a moment of exuberance, knowing no one would be here to cover for me but believing Evan would be further along by now. When we plan, God laughs, as they say. Today, I finally give into the fact that I can't go to Scotland without taking way more Ativan than is healthy. I call Mum and tell her I will have to delay it by a month or so. She is obviously disappointed, but very understanding, as of course she would be. 'Evan comes first,' she says. Yes, he does. It doesn't stop me crying for hours in the bathroom next to Evan's bed. Sometimes, no matter how old you are, you just need your mum.

30 June 2012

On the phone with Mum today she suddenly says à propos of nothing at all, 'Don't you give up, don't start feeling down. You've got to keep your hope.'

We end the call in typical fashion.

Mum: 'Give him a kiss.'

Me: 'Okay (kissing him on the nose).'

Mum: 'Give him another.'

Me: 'Where would you like it?'

Mum: 'On his nose.'

Me: 'I just gave him a kiss on the nose from you.'

Mum: 'Okay, then give him a kiss on the forehead.'

Me: 'Okay.'

Mum: 'Not too hard now.'

Neither of us ever get bored with these conversations.

1 July 2012

I feel so anxious about leaving the hospital today – for the first time since the rapid response – that I have to pop an Ativan just to get out of the hospital. But I have to go home. I have to pay rent, bills, take care of my mail, all the things that don't stop no matter what.

This apartment, it seems a ridiculous expense without Evan in it.

4 July 2012

When the mail arrives there is a card from four friends. They have banded together and sent me some gift cards. It's a lovely surprise. I go out and buy a music speaker for Evan, a very cool pair of commando shorts for him, and two sweaters that will look great on him when the weather gets colder. I take an old iPod of mine, wipe it of its contents, and then set it up in Evan's name and download some lovely children's music.

As soon as I get back to Blythedale I set the speaker and iPod up inside Evan's crib, and let it play for him. We listened to the soundtracks for *Aladdin*, *The Lion King*, and Jack Johnson's *Curious George* soundtrack, which is my favourite of the three; it's mellow and melodic. We keep the music on as I bathe Evan in his big blue tub. Then I give him a long massage – longer than I anticipate as I spill too much massage oil on him. When I realise how much he enjoys it, I resolve to spend more time on massages in the future. He is almost purring.

Later, I write this Facebook post:

4 July 2012

In the first few days of Evan being sick, when it was clear it was going to be a long journey back to recovery, a very compassionate doctor told me to aim ahead at a future date and just see where we would be when we got there, just as a psychological aid in a bad situation. The date he suggested was July 4. Evan and I have spent the day cuddling, listening to music on his new iPod speaker (thanks Anne, Lesley, Tree and Lora, and to Neil and Angela's suggestion of Jack Johnson's *Curious George*) and having a prolonged massage (thanks to the teaching of Rebecca Klinger) (and he got it, I gave it). He is wearing very snazzy clothes (thanks Jackie Frank and Gerry Sugrue) and is surrounded by some very friendly toys (from many, many of you). He's had recent virtual kisses from his aunties Anne and Pauline, and from Clare Grill, Violet Lennon and his Grannie from Glasgow, among others, as well as lovely email wishes from friends, cousins, his mammie's cousins, and even some mammies of friends of his mammie. What more could a boy ask for? We have a very long way to go, but, before and since the nice doctor made his suggestion, we were told many unpleasant 'facts' by well-intentioned doctors, none of which have come to pass. The only thing we can be sure of is that no doctor in the world can predict how smart, strong, athletic or happy Evan is going to be (although the smartest one I have met so far did acknowledge just that). Right now Evan is complaining noisily about three of his first four teeth coming in, and his legs are poking out of the bottom of his pants (because, at ten months, he's a wee monster). He also has a full head of hair, which sits nicely in a Mohawk, and has the cutest wee face in the whole wide world. I know I've missed lots of you in this post, there are so many of you that have helped in so many ways – random emails and texts have been big morale boosts, as have all of your communications with us. My next 'perspective day' is September 3rd – Evan's birthday. Here's hoping for even more great things from the best wee boy in the whole wide world (yer own weans notwithstanding). Happy 4th to all of us.

5 July 2012

I was supposed to be on my way to see my mum today, but instead I spend the day developing a timeline and exhibits for the ACS case.

The expense of the ACS case is really getting to me. I've already spent a fortune (of borrowed money) on lawyers' fees and it seems quite likely that, if we have to go to trial, the final amount will be more than treble that. Treble a fortune! Then there will be the expense of getting an expert. There has also been an ongoing issue that Randi received a bill for Evan's medical records from Columbia University Hospital for over $3,000. They charge 75 cents a page. This is about seven times more than I have ever known anyone to charge for photocopying.

Whenever I get round to making good on these debts it'll be taking money away from Evan and private therapies that might help him. I get that ACS has a job to do, but the emotional strain on me aside, it's cripplingly expensive.

Thinking about all of this gets to be too much so I stop trying to write down everything that happened to Evan and take another Ativan instead.

I have started to realise my Ativan intake has been steadily climbing these past few weeks, but so, of course, has my anxiety. Between the 'Awful and Inappropriate Phone Call', the rapid response, and the stress of ACS's continued role in our lives, I have been finding it very hard to cope. The Ativan does take away the anxiety, but it also tends to flatten my mood. Sometimes, like today, I end up feeling deeply depressed instead.

Now I am so low that even Madison is being nice to me. I prefer it when she's not.

6 July 2012

We are treated to a surprise visit from Ms Pamela Turner this afternoon. She comes in, followed by SW2, who mouths apologies to me behind her back. 'This is Evan,' I say, pointing to him as I place him in his crib. His eyes are a little open as they always are when he sleeps (which is almost always).

'Is he awake? He's not moving,' says Ms Turner in her own inimitable style.

SW2 diplomatically cuts in and says, 'It's difficult to say.' Evan helps us out by moving his hand ever so slightly. We talk for a while about what will happen next.

'It's all up to you,' I tell Ms Turner.

SW2 talks at length in accolades to me – she really lays it on thick.

'Well, I got nothing negative to say about you, it's all positive,' Ms Turner says.

She tells me that she will recommend to the lawyers that they drop the remand, that Evan can come home with me (because there will be a nurse there, it makes it easier) and that she will pay a couple of house visits. I begin to object about being supervised in any way.

'He's my son, I'm his mum, and I haven't done anything wrong.'

Ms Turner is instantly sympathetic.

'No, it's really not like that. It's just a couple visits from me and then we get the judge to dismiss the case. It's simple, it's not a bad thing.'

Well, needless to say, I still don't like any of this, but if this is how it ends then at least this part of things will be over.

I email Randi and tell her what has been said. She replies quickly and says she is suspicious. I tell her not to worry, that I am sure Pamela Turner knows what she is talking about.

7 July 2012

Since the majority of my day is spent sitting down, holding Evan, I spend a lot of time on the internet, including Facebook. It always amazes me that other people are still having normal lives – lives that they are enjoying and want to brag about. Sometimes it hurts me to see their posts about their own children. A good few of them are Evan's age (having a baby makes you befriend other pregnant people). I would shut the account down, but it is my only window on the world right now.

I've felt my spirit slipping again over the last few days. I really just don't have any energy to do anything during the day. I could take a cab into town, or I could just go for a walk, but I have no inclination for anything. Now, even when friends invite me to go out for lunch or dinner, I've been shying away. I don't want to sit in a restaurant talking about sausages when I fear what might happen to Evan without me there. The anxiety just gets too much. And the walk into the hospital, back to his room, not knowing what I will find, has always been terrifying.

The downside though is that, other than holding Evan, there is nothing to do and all day to do it in. The days turn into weeks and now months. My mind and body are atrophying, but my nerves are frayed.

8 July 2012

Nurses Nancy and Kathy are on all weekend – I like them both. They are both in their fifties (I estimate). They are very calm and quiet but they are very observant of Evan. Another thing they do well – better than other nurses – is that when I go home and phone in to see how Evan is they practically cut me off to say, 'He's fine', so I will be put at ease as soon as possible.

Evan's BP is 240/170 this morning. That is beyond ridiculously high. A very young nurse comes in – she is covering for Nancy, who is on break. The young nurse takes her sweet time arranging meds, so much so that I tell her if she doesn't call for a doctor right away I will press the code blue button. This gets a reaction. Kathy comes in to check on her, sees all three of us are upset, takes charge and validates my feelings. This makes me feel better about having been mean to the young one. In turn, of course, once Evan's BP is back to its usual rate I am overcome with guilt for having been mean to the young nurse. It has to be done, though, and I know that if I have to, I will do it again.

10 July 2012

When the nurse came on last night I saw her squeeze the pressure points on Evan's fingernails and get no response. I could feel the darkness creeping over me after that. Half an hour later, as I kissed him goodbye before I went for dinner, I did the same and got a massive reaction from him. The joy of that carried me all the way down to Valhalla and back.

We have a new nurse today. She has been at the hospital for a long time, but we haven't had her before. We start chatting, as I often do with nurses. (It's sociable for me, but I like to think it's good for Evan to hear a conversation around him when I am holding him.) She asks me about the babysitter. It's quite unusual for anyone here to ask me anything about that, and when they do, I always find it quite jarring. But then she turns the conversation to other children that have been at Blythedale.

Apparently there are a lot of abused children in here (I will never get used to Evan being in that category). She tells me about a child, a little girl, who came in with a broken wrist. Her mother was responsible and she lost custody for a while but then the child was given back to her. A few months later the child was back with spinal injuries too. Everyone at Blythedale was furious at ACS that she had been allowed home to her mother in the first place.

I have absolutely no doubt that this was an awful situation, but, as I point out to the nurse, I am the flip side of that: I did nothing to hurt Evan, and love him more than life. But while ACS is waiting to start trying to work out what happened, they have taken custody of him from me. If they feel like it, they can petition to remove my parental rights at any time. They might not succeed, but it gives me chills to think about it.

I can tell this gives the nurse food for thought. The difficulty, of course, is that ACS does need to do what it does if a child is in harm's way. The danger is when they don't do what they need to do, or they don't do it properly, or appropriately, and it causes more harm.

12 July 2012

I come out of therapy this morning and am about to head off to another doctor's appointment, but decide to call the hospital in between the two appointments just to check in. Evan's nurse answers and sounds very upset. She tells me that his blood pressure has fallen sharply and he is very pale. In particular, she says, his extremities are 'mottled'. She tells me she has just called for the doctor. 'He's hanging in there,' she says, with deep concern.

I call a cab, tell the driver my baby is sick, and get back to Evan within fifteen minutes (it's usually a twenty-five-minute trip). I arrive at our room before the doctors arrive (it is lunchtime now, and they are in the canteen, about two minutes down the hall). I pick Evan up. He looks exactly as I had left him. I look at his hands and feet. Yes, his skin is mottled. A lot of us Scots have mottled-looking skin every now and then, especially when the air conditioning is on full blast as it is today. I ask what his blood pressure is. She tells me she just checked it again and it is still 75 over 35. This is not bad for any other baby, but she is used to Evan's blood pressure being sky high. When the doctors arrive they agree with my diagnosis of Scottishness. The poor nurse at least has the grace to look very embarrassed. In fact she looks so mortified that I don't feel the need to chastise her.

Instead I begin to create two mental lists of things medical staff have told me. One is titled 'perceptions' and the other 'truths'. The 'perceptions' list is already very long; the 'truths' list doesn't have many entries so far.

Once everyone leaves the room, I hold Evan and gaze into his big blue eyes and wait, as I always do, for him to come back to me.

15 July 2012

Evan stares at me a lot now. He still can't blink and he can't move his eyes, but he can manage to open them and to fix them on me. He is stepping things up another tiny but precious little notch.

16 July 2012

Randi forwards me an email from Norma's lawyer. It has also been sent to ACS and to Weaver. As the cover letter explains, it contains four letters of recommendation from Norma's prior employers, and the results of a polygraph exam she has passed.

I read the letters of recommendation: they are glowing. This makes me feel a little better about my decision to hire her in the first place.

The polygraph results scare me at first. I try to remember what I'd been taught about them in law school. Eventually I do some research online and am reminded how arbitrary they can be. They measure a physiological reaction, not whether someone is telling the truth. The reaction and the reality are not necessarily the same thing at all. They are so flawed that they are not even admissible in courts in many states, including New York.

I can see from the results that there is already cause for concern about their validity. One of Norma's letters of recommendation talks about a time when she accidentally hurt a child she was looking after and was inconsolable (according to the parent writing it). Yet, during the polygraph she was asked the question, 'Have you ever hurt a child' and she answered no, she had not. The polygraph results didn't pick up on this.

I take another look at the letters of recommendation. Then I go back to work on the timeline and exhibits I have started on, and begin to draft my own cover letter.

I am still working on it late into the evening when the night nurse comes in and tells me to go and get myself a drink, that she will watch Evan for me.

As I sit at the bar in the Cabin, alone, as usual, I become aware of something that has been staring me in the face all this time: in all these months, Norma and I have been pitched against each other by ACS. I have been focusing far too much on her. In actual fact, whatever Norma did or did not do to Evan, it does not tell the entire story.

Norma and I took Evan to two doctors, one in the hospital in January, and then, after that, to his paediatrician. After we had moved to Blythedale, Dr Brown had written me a letter explaining her findings of the January hospitalisation. She was quite clear. She wrote that the hospital doctor released Evan without doing a CT scan and that this was in error. He also missed information in one of Evan's blood tests results – established evidence Evan had had some seizure activity before being admitted to hospital. If that doctor had done his job properly, perhaps Evan could have been put on anti-seizure medication.

If he had carried out a CT scan, he would surely have seen some evidence of the seizure, but I'm not convinced he would have found evidence of shaking. I assume he looked in Evan's eyes when he examined him, because doctors always do. But there was nothing noted to say that Evan had bleeding in his retinas at that time, which is a significant component of SBS. And then there was Evan's regular paediatrician. He was shown a video which every other doctor tells me clearly shows Evan having a seizure. But he failed to diagnose it as one because he didn't know that seizures do not require repetitive movements of the limbs.

I know that we were very unlucky in finding not one but two doctors who couldn't diagnose seizure activity despite clear evidence of it. However, neither of these doctors suspected SBS. If it had been going on since January (as Dr Brown believes), surely one or both of them would have noticed retinal bleeding?

Another piece of the puzzle is that Randi told me recently that ACS has now established that Evan was definitely shaken, but that there is no evidence to say he was shaken more than twice. So much for the young doctor on the first night saying it had happened multiple times. He should never have been allowed out of his lab. He certainly didn't have the social or professional skills to speak with an anxious parent. And now it's clear he didn't even have the medical expertise to convey the results accurately.

I suppose, with a clear head, I can conclude three things:

1. Both doctors (the paediatrician, and the doctor at the first hospitalisation) were negligent in not realising Evan was having seizures.

2. Norma shook Evan twice. But it's not unreasonable to believe that she did so when he was seizing to try and get him out of the seizure. That is incredibly dangerous and foolish, but it is not child abuse.

3. For every doctor that has an opinion, there is another doctor that can contradict that opinion. Now they are saying it happened twice. Maybe at some point they will say it didn't happen at all.

What is really concerning about all this is the difference in punishment. Those two doctors deserve a malpractice action. If there is one, and they are found guilty, their insurance company will make a payout. Then the doctors will complain (like every other doctor) that their insurance premiums will increase. They will likely not applaud themselves for the incredible medical expenses their negligence caused. That will be the end of it for them. They won't go to jail, and they won't lose their medical licences.

If Norma's role is what I think it is, and she shook Evan in a panic at his seizing, she has been grossly negligent too. But she faces child abuse charges in family court, and might even face criminal charges later. She could go to jail, as well as being labelled a child abuser.

And me? I could lose custody of Evan on the basis of nothing whatsoever. I've already had to spend a huge amount to defend myself and the stress has been unbearable.

ACS has run away with this case, and entirely in the wrong direction. But the ACS charges are so severe and serious that they have turned my head. I really need to step back and try and work things out for myself. I'm not so sure Norma has played anything other than a bit part in all of this.

17 July 2012

I change Evan's tracheostomy tube for the first time today (I had only ever changed the ties before). It is both immensely easy and exceptionally terrifying. All you have to do is prepare the new tube, get the new ties ready, have the Ambu bag handy, and then, in a swift movement, pull the old tube out and stick the new one in and attach the vent hose to it. Then you secure the ties around his neck. After that your stomach swirls and your head aches and you take quite some time to get over what you just had to do to your baby. But you have to do it.

Once it is all done I feel superhuman.

18 July 2012

I feel like a total idiot.

I thought I was being smart and I booked myself in for a polygraph test. I should have known better; I know they are unreliable. They only measure reactions, and reactions can be explained by many things, not just honesty or dishonesty, but I really wanted to try it.

To prepare, I look up a few articles on the internet, including one about what to do to prepare for a polygraph. It basically says don't do anything: if you read and understand too much about how the polygraph works then you will compromise its effectiveness. So I shut down the computer and don't look into it any further.

The test day arrives and I call a taxi to take me to the office of the polygraph examiner. It turns out it isn't actually his office. It is a conference centre at Westchester Airport, a tiny airport that I didn't even know existed until now. It's an overcast day, with a bit of rain. I sit in the waiting area, having arrived a good twenty minutes early. I watch a family disembark from a small private plane, dressed in very summery clothes, and start to turn blue as they wait for a shuttle bus to collect them and take them to their final destination. Seems to be a poorly planned trip all round for them. Eventually another small plane touches down. A middle-aged man gets out. He walks down the portable staircase that has been delivered to his tiny plane's door. He exchanges a few words with the ground crew and then walks into the waiting area. He sees me, alone on the couches, and introduces himself: he is the polygraph examiner.

He asks me to wait there while he gets the room ready. A few minutes later he comes back and tells me to follow him. We go into a long, dimly lit conference room with a window that looks onto the tarmac. We can see his plane. We chit-chat for a bit. He tells me he has flown from western New York and it has taken him a couple of hours; that it probably cost him around $250 to make the flight; and that he conducts many of his tests in airport conference rooms like the one we are in. He seems amiable.

He asks me why I am taking a polygraph. I tell him everything. I explain that Norma has already taken one and that she has passed it. I tell him how she has managed to get past one question, which, by her own evidence, she should have failed. I hand him the copy of her report. 'I know this guy,' he says, pointing to the name on the letterhead of the report. 'Yeah, he's got some real shady practices.' I tell him all the issues I have thought of already.

'Yeah, I can write you a report and say all the things this guy has done wrong with this here test, and I can see a few things already, just looking at it.'

'Okay, great – how much will you charge?'

'$250,' he says.

Well, gosh, that's just enough to cover your transportation here today, I think. I agree, thinking I have won a watch with this guy. The truth will out at last! Then we set to, getting my own test underway.

He explains that he will hook me up with a monitor around my chest, to measure my heart rate, and a monitor on my palm and on some of my fingers, which will measure how much I perspire, and will also measure my heart rate. After that, he will ask me five questions. Each one of these questions will be embedded in a group of other questions, all of which are 'control' questions, to which my answers are true and agreed upon by both of us (for example, 'Is it raining?' 'Yes'). The measure of my reaction to answering the control questions will provide a means to measure my responses to the important questions. We will agree what each and every question is in advance so that I won't be surprised by anything. (Surprise would cause a response in me that would register with the machines and skew the results.) To make sure there are no other conditions that will affect my responses he asks me if I slept well last night, if I am on any medication ('Yes, lots'), if I have any other concerns, and if I am menstruating ('No, but thanks for asking').

The control questions are strange.

'Have you ever told a lie?'

'Well, yes,' I say, 'I think everyone has told a lie at some point in their life.'

'Well, most people would answer no to that question,' he says.

'But that's just not realistic,' I tell him.

Then I tell him how I was in the closet for years and told many lies to hide being gay, and how it's now extremely important to me that I am as truthful as possible in everything I say and do, but that there are always little white lies that I catch myself saying (although, when I do, I always try to correct them). I impress on him that everyone lies at some point; it's human nature.

'Being in the closet doesn't count because you were protecting yourself,' he says, clearly hoping to move on.

'Yes, but if Norma is lying it is to protect herself, too. It's the same for anyone who feels the need to lie in a polygraph, I presume.'

He is getting agitated.

'Do you recall anything else you've ever lied about?' he says, running his hand through his hair.

Put on the spot, I try to think of an example.

'Well, I remember when I was six years old and my mum sent me in to a shop to get her a packet of cigarettes and she told me not to buy candy but I did and I hid it in my waistband, and when we got home, she asked me if I had bought candy and I said no, and then she lifted my T-shirt to show all the candy sticking out of my waistband. I very clearly remember her telling me how disappointed she was that I had lied to her.'

'Okay,' he says, 'so we'll incorporate that. The question will be, "Other than one time when you were six years old, have you ever told a lie?"'

Jeez, I can think of more, but I am starting to feel a bit of pressure from him to get things going. Anyway, we clearly aren't on the same page as to what it is to tell a lie – not according to him anyway. So I say okay, and on we go.

'Have you ever physically harmed anyone? Don't include fist-fights you got into as a child,' he adds quickly.

'Well, there was this one time I was in DC for a friend's wedding. A few of us were sitting in the lobby of the hotel we were staying in. We got chatting to a couple of doctors who were in town for a convention. One of them didn't like the way my friend was totally trouncing him in a political argument so he lifted up her skirt. She was sitting down and she was shocked by it. I was standing next to him, so I just reached up and slapped him on the back of his head and told him to behave himself. Another friend of ours called security and when they came, the doctor said, 'I was just assaulted.' All my friends stood up for me, of course; pointed out the doctor had just committed an indecent assault. Another doctor stepped in and hustled his friend into an elevator and he disappeared. The second doctor came back down a while later and apologised for him. Does that count?' I ask.

'No, just say no to that question,' is the reply.

I don't really focus on the rest of the control questions as I am still thinking about people saying they don't tell lies. He goes over the questions – the substantive ones – that he is going to ask me. Have I ever hit Evan? Have I ever thrown Evan? Have I ever dropped Evan? Have I ever hurt Evan? Have I ever shaken Evan? I have to stop him in the middle of this and explain how upset I am getting at the questions.

'Every time you say those questions it makes me feel really emotional. Not even at the thought of me being accused of it, but that anyone would do any of those things to him.'

I am close to tears.

'Well, did you drop or shake him or throw him?'

'No, I didn't!' I said.

'So say no when you're asked and if you're telling the truth the machine will show it,' he says, looking down and onto the next part of the test.

'But I have hurt him,' I say. 'I have to pinch his fingers to see if he responds – if he does then that means he has felt pain. And he was suctioned at birth – that was my decision and it scratched and bruised his head a bit. And one time when I was kissing him my watchstrap caught his head and he screamed. I felt awful and I didn't mean it, but yes, I did hurt him.'

'Okay, none of that counts,' he declares, looking down studiously at his laptop again.

We get started on the test. By this time I have already been here for about an hour and the room is cold (the air conditioning is still on despite the cooler temperatures outside). I feel a bit strung out and wish I had brought an Ativan with me (I didn't because I knew that would skew the results). He hooks me up to the wires and tells me to sit facing the door, away from him. Then he starts asking the questions. Each time he asks one of the five 'real' questions, 'Have you ever hurt Evan?' I answer forcefully, 'No.' He tells me to stop doing that.

'Just answer in a normal voice or you'll skew the test.'

But there is no 'normal voice' in which to answer these questions. Each time he asks each question I have the same feelings of sadness and horror, really, that this is what happened to Evan. I have managed to get through an awful lot of this situation by ignoring this reality, so it certainly doesn't feel good to be hearing it now. I can feel my heart rate increase on my own – I don't need his machine to tell me about it.

Once we are done he unhooks me and goes back to studying his laptop. He doesn't want to catch my eye. I leave and take a cab back to the hospital.

Today, I get an email from the polygraph guy.

'The results were not favourable and I am unable to rule you out as a suspect in Evan's case.'

I have been expecting that. I know that my responses were more pronounced when I heard those horrible questions.

I resume the polygraph research I had abandoned in the interests of purity of the test. There is so much material on the internet about the unreliability of polygraphs. I read about a father accused of incest with his daughter. Both of them vehemently deny it. The father's test results say he is lying, although the daughter's results say she is telling the truth. The father describes afterwards how upset he had been to hear questions about whether he had sex with his daughter. I can completely understand how he could respond so profoundly when asked if he had hurt his child (and in a horrendous way). There is example after example, article after article, about why polygraphs don't work.

I wish I had been more cautious about taking a polygraph test. I wish I had done more research and focused instead only on their unreliability. Now I have nothing. I can't exactly argue, 'Norma's test results can't be reliable because I failed mine and I know I didn't do this, so, as she passed hers, she must be guilty.'

Also, of course, I can't even use the examiner's report in which he criticises Norma's polygraph examiner's techniques quite strongly. If I do, and ACS calls him in to answer questions about his report, they will be sure to ask how he knows me. 'Oh, she came in for a polygraph.' 'Did she now… that's interesting… and what were the results?'

19 July 2012

A nurse asks me when my court date is. It really rattles me to think that everyone here knows about it – and who knows what they are thinking? Maybe that's why Madison is always so hostile to me? Anyway, it feels humiliating and degrading, just like the rest of the ACS process.

20 July 2012

I have to come back to the city for the final hearing date of my final case as a lawyer. Evan looks well when I leave him this morning. He is nice and limber inasmuch as his left elbow can bend pretty well, even if his right arm still refuses to. His blood pressure is a little better. He is even making his guttural little noises, which I love more than anything.

Nonetheless, I still have enough anxiety remaining as I leave him that I have to load up on Ativan to make the trip to Manhattan. For the most part, I enjoy the hearing. I manage to impeach the chief witness for the defence and do a little bit of showboating along the way. All the stuff you imagine doing as you sit through all those law-school classes.

And then it's over.

As I travel back to Westchester on the train I get my usual blast of anxiety, which makes me realise that, no matter how much I will miss it, I am a million miles away from being capable of resuming my law career right now.

I get back to the hospital to find that, after four months of us living here, Blythedale has finally worked out that I've been sneaking my laundry in with Evan's all this time. His clothes have been delivered, freshly laundered. Mine have been carefully extracted from our dirty laundry bag, placed in a paper bag and put right back into our cupboard, still dirty.

21 July 2012

One of the nursing assistants comes by for a chat (they are usually a lot more friendly than the nurses). She tells me that she has a second job at a long-term care facility nearby. The patients there are all under two years old, and most of them were born with their conditions. And there they are, consigned to a life in an institution. No matter how beautiful some of the facilities can be (and Blythedale and Elizabeth Seton certainly are), surely none can compare with being in a loving home? But, according to the nursing assistant, a lot of the parents don't stay involved with their children once they get admitted. She was far from judgemental, saying that they often just can't deal with the situation.

I suppose there's an emotional attachment that all carers have to carefully balance with their professionalism. As a young lawyer I put far too much emotional effort into some cases. I was at real risk of burning out. As I got more experienced, the energy I used was professional, and far less emotional. I'm not sure if that had any impact on the results I started to get, but it certainly affected my stress levels in a good way.

I've seen some nurses who clearly don't have any emotional involvement, particularly at the ICU, and that's probably their coping mechanism. But at Blythedale there really does seem to be an extra air of care around the nursing staff and therapists who look after Evan.

22 July 2012

When I come in from dinner tonight, the two nurses are sitting in their oval booth, at Evan's pod, outside the children's rooms, as usual. One is facing her computer screen and me. The other is facing away from her screen and, therefore, also facing me, but sitting a few feet behind the first. As I walk in, the first nurse says to me, 'How are you?' The second nurse, not realising who spoke, says to me, 'Good, thanks.'

23 July 2012

I think I have a new angle on what happened to Evan. I've written a letter to ACS explaining it. I have included a timeline of events and a binder of exhibits. It's taken me several weeks to get all of this together — a task that as a fully functioning lawyer might have taken me an afternoon.

160 W. 71st Street, Apt 6B
New York, NY 10023
(917) 848 8736

July 23, 2012
Weaver
NYC Administration for Children's Service

<u>Re: Evan Schwarz</u>

I Believe in Evan

Dear [ACS and Weaver]:

I write in my capacity as Evan Schwarz's mother. Regardless of the pending action against me, the prevailing issue, as I am sure you agree, is Evan's health and wellbeing, both now and in the future. To that end, I have a pressing need to know what happened to cause his injuries. If there is any chance at all that this can be definitively established by your investigations then I impress on you to do what you can. I respectfully submit this letter as an aid to your investigations, and in the hope that you will leave no stone unturned to give my family closure in this matter.

I have briefly read the letters of recommendation for Norma Leonce, and can tell you that I have absolutely no argument with the sentiment contained in each of them. I have always known Norma to be kind and caring, and I would not have let her babysit Evan if I did not have full faith and trust in her to take care of him properly.

I do feel, however, that Norma found herself in an impossibly stressful situation as regards the episodes (so far apparently unexplained) that led to Evan not breathing and, at times, turning blue. I did not appreciate this until the one and only time I witnessed him turning blue: in June, and at Blythedale hospital. I was holding him in my arms when his vent began to alarm. Fortunately there was a nurse standing next to us and she helped me check all the connections, but we couldn't find anything disconnected. Then I looked back at Evan and his eyelids and mouth were turning blue. The 'code blue' button was pressed and I carefully placed him on the bed, where he got even more blue. Although he was instantly attended to by doctors, nurses and respiratory therapists, and was revived within seconds, I was hysterical and inconsolable from the experience. I can only imagine how stressful it was for Norma to have to deal with this on at least two occasions.

I have never been able to reconcile my knowledge of Norma's caring character with the idea that she intentionally injured Evan. I have personal knowledge, however, that she tends to panic in stressful situations. For example, and as referenced in the 'Timeline' document (submitted hereto), on the first occasion Evan turned blue (January 18, 2012), Norma called me at work, screaming, and barely understandable. On that occasion, I had to call an ambulance (in her stead) because, as it later emerged, she had been too upset to recall the address of the apartment. (I immediately pinned all important details, including the address, to a wall in the apartment.) When I arrived at the apartment, Norma explained that she had performed CPR on Evan. She explained that she had turned him onto his front and used the heel of her hand to stimulate his back. As I recently learned when I received CPR training, these actions are supposed to be employed when a child is choking, not when a child cannot breathe: although Norma is qualified in CPR, in a moment of crisis she chose the wrong technique. Just days later, on January 24, 2012, Norma called me at work, again, and again was screaming and barely understandable due to her emotions. After this occasion I installed a landline, in the hope that this would make it easier to understand her if she called in heightened emotion again. Again, as I did after the first occasion, I spoke to her and explained how important it was to keep calm if the situation arose again.

All of these incidences, when measured alongside my understanding of how frightening Evan's breath-holding and 'blue' episodes are, lead me to imagine that, when Norma was confronted by these situations she was unable to remain rational and, perhaps acting in a manner intended only to revive him, chose the wrong technique and in fact shook him. While this, of course, is entirely the wrong reaction and, if true, has led to immeasurable harm to Evan, I do find it plausible, in light of all the circumstantial evidence.

I have read Norma's polygraph test results, albeit with scepticism, given the unreliability of such tests, and noting, of course, their resultant inadmissibility in New York courts. This limitation notwithstanding, I am struck by a glaring inconsistency between the test taken and one of the employer references submitted. Ms Amber D. Harris states that Norma accidentally hurt her son by pinching his leg with the strap of his stroller, leading to him sustaining a small bruise. As Ms Harris recalls, this incident greatly upset Norma, despite the minimal injury. However, when asked the questions, 'Have you ever harmed an infant?' and 'Have you ever been involved in harming an infant?' Norma replied in the negative, and no deception was found. Such apparent innocence of the inaccuracy of her response surely indicates that she does not equate her accidental, or even incidental, injury of an infant with 'causing harm'. Clearly 'harm' was caused to Ms Harris's child, and clearly, by her own admission, Norma either 'harmed' him or was 'involved' in harming him. I can only conclude that Norma understood this question to require deliberate harm only. This would of course explain Norma's denial of having harmed Evan, even if she did shake him in an effort to revive him, but without malicious intent.

I therefore request that you pursue this possibility in your investigations. As you must be aware, I have been forced to expend considerable sums in the action against me. It is neither possible nor reasonable that I should incur the expense of pursuing the same investigation that your offices are established to pursue. Furthermore, if Norma did indeed shake Evan to revive him, but is not in fact aware that these actions caused him such extensive harm, it is vital that she be informed and educated in this regard so as to avoid the same thing happening to another child in her future care. With both these aspects in mind, I suggest that you take the following direct and indirect measures to establish the truth:

1. Enquire of Norma as to whether she shook Evan in an attempt to revive him;
2. Subpoena the full names and addresses of all of Norma's past and present employers, including the employer immediately prior to her retention by me, a lady by the name of Debbie;
3. Enquire as to the identity of the child and parent who had a seizure when in Norma's care (as to her representations to me on January 18, 2012).

Finally, I request that you fully investigate all other possible causes of Evan's injury. I am aware that there exists a medical point of view which indicates that the existence of old blood (which Evan's CT scan showed) might not be indicative of prior acts of shaking, but, in fact, of a neurological issue, such as a stroke, for example. I understand that Cornell Hospital did not find retinal bleeding (during Evan's 1/18/12 hospitalisation), and, of course, am all too aware that they neglected to perform a CT scan. In light of that, perhaps this medical theory should be employed. Once again, I do not have the resources to pursue this avenue at this time, but I do expect your offices to do so, given your remit in this matter.

Blythedale

Thank you for your consideration of these suggestions.

Very Truly Yours,

Elise Schwarz

24 July 2012

I sleep until 11.10am this morning. I hate sleeping so late in the hospital. With all the nurses, therapists and doctors, it basically feels like you're sleeping in someone's workplace.

I have to go back into the city again, this time to Brooklyn, where I have a Brownstone townhouse that I co-own with a friend. We've had it for seven years, and have been renting it out. We bought it a year before the peak of the housing boom but, like so many others, refinanced it right at the peak. It probably still hasn't reached its potential, but with all of my mounting debts I really have no option but to sell it and take what I can for it.

While I am sitting on the stoop in the scorching heat, waiting for the broker to appear, I get an email from Randi. I am aware she was going to talk to Lubin and Weaver today, after she sent them my timeline and cover letter. I have been waiting for contact from her and am really hoping for some good news. Instead her email simply reads, 'We need an expert.'

In this short sentence I know that the lawyers won't budge; that my good report card from Ms Turner has not been considered; nor have the documents I had meticulously prepared and explained. Trial is looming. I'll be even more in debt. But worse than any of that, I'm scared I will lose Evan.

I let rip with a volley of emails to Randi. Four in a row, each with more swear words than the one before. Randi is a good person to do that to. She doesn't shrink from profanity, far from it, and she can also soak up my emotions quite well (or she wouldn't be so blunt with me). After I was done she emailed to say that nothing has actually changed, we are in the same position as yesterday.

Yes, except that yesterday I had a bit of hope that today the position would change.

I distract myself this evening by getting my hair done in a real hair salon. I even get it coloured. I've been dyeing it myself these past few months, but I find out today that I only have a knack for doing the parts I can see in the mirror. The hairdresser gives me a quizzical look as he holds a mirror so I can see the two inches of solidly white hair streaking down the middle of the back of my head. I assume, optimistically, that it's been hidden by the ponytail that I wear relentlessly.

25 July 2012

I sleep late again, this time in my own bed at home, luxuriously splaying out into a starfish for much of the night. I'm usually balancing on about a foot and a half of my rock solid little sofa-turned-bed at the hospital, so it's a treat.

I get back to find Evan looking lovely, and not a worry on him. I sit with him for a long time. Suddenly, entirely out of the blue, the vent starts beeping. The nurse on duty doesn't get a warning alarm at her desk, so I have to call her several times. This exacerbates my anxiety. When she comes in I have Evan on the bed and his chest has clearly stopped rising and falling. He isn't getting any breaths at all. The nurse hits the rapid response button and, as usual, within seconds the room is full of doctors and nurses.

I take myself out of the way, and end up with my back to the wall cupboards, staring at the scene. I am aware of one nurse asking me if I am okay: I feel faint.

'Quick, sit down,' she says, although I haven't answered her.

I make the two steps it takes to get to my bed, but as I sit down, suddenly my hands cramp up and become like claws at the end of my arms. At first I can't move them, then I can't even feel them. The loss of sensation is spreading upwards, towards my elbows.

'You're hyperventilating,' says a doctor.

My neck starts cramping up too. Someone runs in with a paper bag. It is the best they can find, but it was one of the very large ones that they use for laundry (not mine any more, of course). So the nurse does what she can and puts my entire head into it and tells me to breathe with her.

It takes a while, but I eventually manage to calm down, get the sensation back in the bits of my body that have lost it and, of course, burst into tears. They can't be nicer to me. One of them even manages to say, 'I like your hair.'

It turns out Evan had a plug in his tube, which is quite common and really simple to fix (either by suctioning it out or by changing the tube). So he was fine almost immediately, but the doctor and nurses spent about twenty more minutes attending to me. Eventually, I am calm enough to hold Evan again. He gives me a reward, moving his eyes across my face.

A few hours later, I go to a meditation group organised by the hospital. It is well-timed, given the events of the day. There are six of us, all mothers, all with very sick children. We each introduce ourselves and tell our stories. The tears flow.

One mother's teenage son was very badly burned in an accident a year and a half ago and has been in here almost ever since. Another's twelve-year-old boy was injured in a car accident two months ago. The three of us share the unenviable status of having been told, several times, that our children are not likely to survive. Two other mothers have children that are recuperating from operations, which are not life threatening, but obviously stressful nonetheless. The sixth woman has a three-month-old baby who was born with an underdeveloped cerebellum. No one has any idea how she will progress.

It is remarkably helpful hearing about other parents' experiences. We are all quite candid about how gruelling our lives have become. One mother talks about how she often gets asked how she can hold up so well.

'I could roll about the floor screaming and wailing, I suppose, and I have done that, but I can't do it all day every day – it's been a year and a half already, that's a long time to scream and wail.'

I suddenly don't feel quite so isolated. Especially not when the two mothers of the more critical children start comically comparing 'code blue' stories of their offspring.

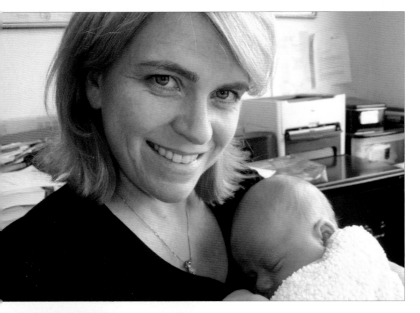

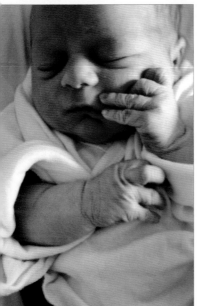

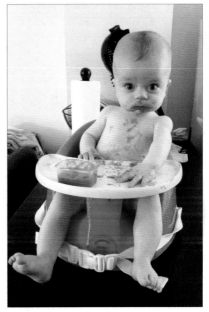

Above: Evan and me in my office in Manhattan. He's just a few weeks old.

Below left: Evan's second day, taken in the hospital.

Below right: Carrots! Evan loved carrots, although he preferred peas.

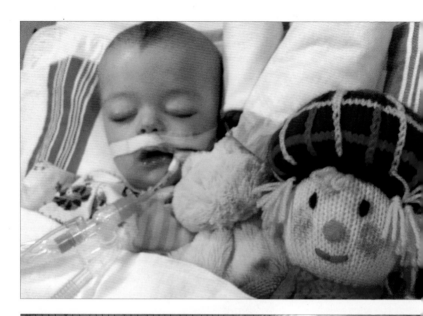

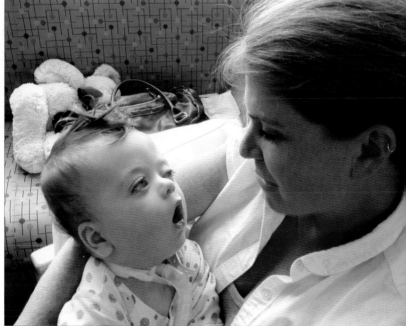

Above: This is Evan, a few weeks into his hospitalisation.

Below: Evan on his first birthday. We are in Blythedale. The couch in the background is also my bed.

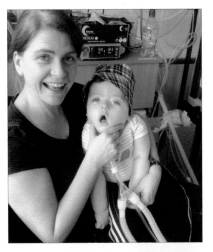

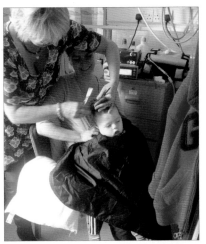

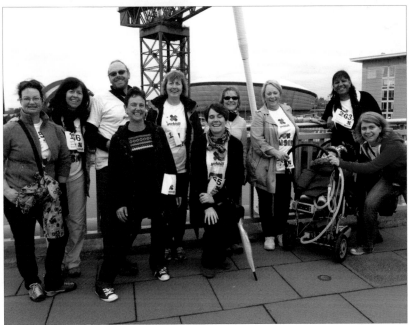

Above left: Evan in Yorkhill children's hospital. We are just back from a lovely walk around the West End of Glasgow.

Above right: Evan's first haircut.

Below: Some of the Schwarz relatives in town for the family reunion take part in a sponsored walk for Yorkhill. The Finnieston Quay and the new Hydro stadium are in the background.

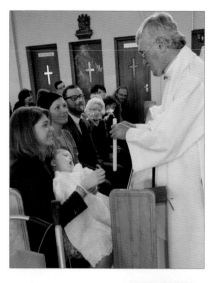

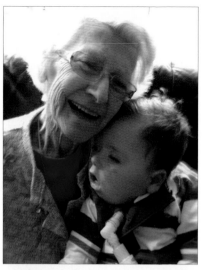

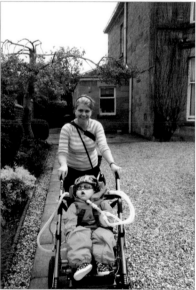

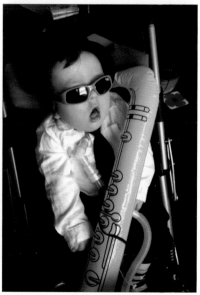

Above left: Evan's christening. Violet and Neil are to our left, and Father Michael is officiating.

Above right: Evan and his granny having a cuddle.

Below left: Evan and I are off for a walk in the park. The holly tree is in the background, looking worse for wear.

Below right: Halloween 2013!

Then we meditate. I'm not good at that kind of thing at the best of times, but especially not tonight – I still have too much adrenaline coursing through my veins from the hyperventilation. I sit with my eyes closed and my mind racing.

26 July 2012

I was talking with Angela B today and she asked me if she could do anything for me. I told her to come to New York, half-joking, half-hoping. Within a few hours she had booked another week's trip at the beginning of August. That gives me something to look forward to.

1 August 2012

Terrible sleep last night. Having horrendous dreams or skirting consciousness all night long. I wake up laden with anxiety about the ACS case, trying desperately to think of a plan, and coming up with nothing again and again.

A whole lot of cousins have started to arrive in New York for my cousin's son's wedding on Long Island this Saturday. Evan and I had a lovely visit from my cousin Pat yesterday. She lives in the Scottish Highlands and brought Evan a pair of slippers shaped like the Loch Ness monster and a pair of Celtic Football Club pyjamas. She also brought a gift for the nurses: a box of shortbread. I don't think that's something that's done here, although it's very common in Scotland. I had hoped for a piece myself but they had disappeared by the time I got back from walking Pat out of the building.

I Believe in Evan

Today Pat's sister, my cousin Con, visited with her husband, Peter. They live in England. They brought some Marks and Spencer's baby clothes for Evan (excellent quality) and some nice bath soaps for me. I'm always concerned how people will react when they see Evan. It's led to me rejecting offers of visits in the past. But if any of these visitors felt any sense of shock they certainly didn't show it and it couldn't have been more lovely to see them.

2 August 2012

Angela B arrives today – yay! She is to head straight to my apartment. The doorman will give her a spare key. She and I will meet there around 2pm.

I leave the hospital early, having had a run in with Madison again, this time over painkillers. Evan's heart rate is very high and he is sweating which, we have already agreed, is probably an indication he is having teething pain.

'If I give him painkillers now, I won't have anything to give him later,' she argues.

'If you give it to him now, you won't need to give it to him later,' I counter.

She is unmoved by my logic but I am tired of her already and tell her, 'I am not going to beg you for painkillers. I'm his mother and I am telling you he needs them.'

He gets them. I hold him for half an hour or so and he is calm and sleeping. Then I leave.

I have terrible anxiety walking down to the train station. I feel my chest tighten and my breath shorten. I pop an Ativan halfway through the graveyard and calm down. It is quite scary how well that drug works.

After catching up on some errands, I get back to my apartment, where I can see I have just missed Angela B. The internet is still showing on the computer screen and the straightening irons are still warm. (I should have been a detective.) While I wait for her to return, I pop downstairs to the doctors' surgery (another reason why my apartment is in a great location), where I have an appointment to check whether my chest tightening is an issue. I have to explain my situation to yet another doctor. In the end, her advice is simple: keep taking the Ativan. At least this reduces my 'pill-popper's guilt' a little.

When Angela and I finally meet up it's wonderful to see her. We chat for hours. As I have intended to do, I tell her all about the ACS case. She is very calm, and says reassuring things to me. She tells me she has heard of this kind of situation before, in Scotland too, where everyone present comes under suspicion. It is a relief to not be keeping the secret from her any more.

4 August 2012

THE WEDDING

We arrived on Long Island yesterday. It's a four-hour train trip from Westchester, as you have to go via Manhattan and change from Grand Central to Penn Station.

This morning I call the hospital (for the twentieth time since

I have left) and am told that Evan has been given a dose of Ativan because the nurse thought he was having a seizure. As we know by now, Evan doesn't have seizures. As we also know, Ativan doesn't mix well with the other medicines he is on. I am very concerned. She reassures me that he seems to be doing fine now.

I get ready and meet the rest of the wedding guests in the lobby of the hotel as planned. Also as planned, Angela B heads off to a nearby mall. She doesn't know anyone other than me and is content to check out Long Island while I am at the wedding.

I pile into the rental mini van along with the rest of the wedding guests and we head to the church. It's already very hot, and the kilts and dress attire are looking set to start wilting.

Once we get to the church, I wait outside as everyone files into their respective sides. Then I call the hospital again. This time the on-call doctor gets on the line and tells me he is worried about Evan. I ask if I should come back, but he says he doesn't think it's necessary.

I enter the church, apologising profusely as I pass by the bride and her family, who are waiting in the entranceway to proceed.

The wedding is beautiful. I worry about Evan the entire ceremony. When everyone gets outside and has serenaded the newly-weds to their waiting car, I call the hospital again. I am told things still aren't great, but no worse. This really doesn't make me feel much better.

We arrive at the reception location, a beautiful yacht club overlooking the water. As much as I don't want to cast a shadow on the happy couple's day in any way, I really can't contain myself and so I quickly make my excuses to a few of the cousins (all of whom know what is going on and are very concerned). I call a taxi and then go and stand in the car park, waiting.

Con's husband, Peter, comes out to keep me company. He can see I am upset, even through my sunglasses. 'It's all part of the battle,' he says, consolingly. He offers me his pint of beer, which I take, and finish. He takes $50 from his sporran and gives it to me to pay for the cab that has just arrived. I get in and speed off back to the hotel to get my things.

I get a call from the hospital when I am in the cab. The doctor tells me he feels that Evan's condition is deteriorating inasmuch as his blood pressure has dropped dangerously low. He tells me he is referring him to the ICU in nearby Westchester Medical Center. I am already on my way back, which is the only positive.

Back at the hotel, Angela B isn't anywhere to be found. It's still only 1pm and she's probably at the mall. She doesn't have a working mobile. I send her an email, leave my iPad out for her and leave a note on top, telling her I am already on my way back to Westchester and to check her emails.

I go back downstairs where the taxi driver is waiting for me and we race to the train station, where I quickly get a train back to the city.

Two cabs, two trains, a subway and almost four hours later I reach Blythedale. When I get there, the ambulance has only just arrived and the paramedics are in the process of preparing Evan for the journey to the ICU. I ask them what they think is wrong and it becomes clear that no one is really sure. It's also clear, to me at least, that he isn't any different from when I left him.

I raise the issue of the Ativan with the paramedics and ask them whether, with all the blood pressure medication he is already on, the combination is what's caused the drop. They say they don't know, but they have to take him anyway.

There are always risks in transporting a vent-dependent patient. The vent can be moved, so long as it's done properly, but what if the ambulance is involved in an accident? There is also the effect of being outside – it can alter blood pressure and heart rate, which in turn can affect the patient's health. I really don't want Evan moved unnecessarily, but with that said, I don't feel that I can second-guess the doctor.

Eventually – a full seven hours after the doctor's call telling me of the emergency situation – we arrive in the ER of Westchester Medical Center (which is a ten-minute walk from Blythedale, even without pavements). Evan is hooked up to all the same machines as usual, as well as a few extra ones. The ER doctor comes in and examines him and I have to tell the entire story of what happened to him all over again.

'Are ACS involved?' he asks.

'Oh yes,' I reply, although I don't give him more details than that, and he doesn't ask.

It is clear from the monitors that Evan's blood pressure is now back to its usual reading. His oxygen levels are good and his heart rate is normal too. After a while the ER doctor tells me he doesn't know exactly why Evan has been transferred to the ER. We are taken upstairs to the ICU and Evan is settled for a second time. The ICU doctor comes in and examines him. He doesn't have any idea why Evan is here either.

At about 8pm my mobile rings and shows my home number on caller ID: it is Angela B. She hadn't been able to get the iPad to work and had no other way of contacting me so she made the journey back to the city, terrified as to what might have happened to Evan, and only now able to contact me. I explain what I can and tell her Evan is fine. We arrange to meet in the Cabin a few hours later.

When we meet, we are both frazzled and emotionally spent. It turns out to be one of the funniest evenings ever. We have both been running on high emotions for most of the day, and are both extremely relieved that things haven't been as bad as it seemed they might be at one point. So we sit at the bar, relaxed and drinking beer, and put the world to rights.

Angela decides that as we have an average age of forty-four, that's the age we will both use.

'See, people of our age, forty-four…'

'But you're forty-seven and I'm forty-one.'

'Yes. So on average we're forty-four…'

She manages this with an entirely straight face. A few drinks and similar conversation later, we end up in hysterics. We laugh so much that I actually feel self-conscious at showing that side of me in the Cabin.

6 August 2012

I stayed at the ICU with Evan these last two nights. Yesterday another new shift of doctors, nurses and respiration therapists arrived and I had to explain the situation all over again as I had done on day one. How I hate talking about what happened to Evan.

One of the difficulties of Evan being transported is that he now has to be on one of Westchester Medical Hospital's stationary vents, not on the portable one that he is used to. Each vent is different, and vent settings always have to be adjusted to get them just right.

I notice that one of the options on the new vent, 'CPAP', is lit up when it wasn't lit up on the portable vent at Blythedale. I ask the doctor about it but he says it is fine and doesn't elaborate. I know better than to take anyone's word for anything any more so, when a nurse comes in, I ask her about it.

'That doesn't matter,' she says.

'Are you sure? I always thought that it did.'

'No, it doesn't.'

'Well, wait a minute, why is it an option if it doesn't matter?'

She loses patience. 'You're not understanding me,' she says.

'No, obviously I am not understanding you,' I say, irritated.

She throws her hands in the air, says, 'I'm not working with this baby', turns on her heel and storms out. I can't believe it.

The other nurse, the one who is actually assigned to Evan, starts to apologise. I turn to face the window, trying not to react. Was it really important to that nurse to make things even more unpleasant? She comes back in and says she is sorry. By now I am biting back the tears and keep focused on the window. She leaves again. Thankfully I don't see her after that, and Evan's nurse continues to be pleasant enough to me.

Evan is eventually allowed back to Blythedale, having

received no treatment whatsoever at the ICU, because none has been needed. It is something of a comfort to get back to our usual surroundings, even though I am still quite annoyed by the whole experience.

10 August 2012

The rest of Angela B's stay is without incident, and when she leaves today, I am sorry to see her go. I have only just waved goodbye to her at the corner of 71st and Broadway when I receive an email from Randi with the ACS case file attached. It includes all the notes of the caseworkers. I decide not to read it; it will be too painful to revisit the events of February, and I don't see the point in upsetting myself when Angela's visit has left me in a pleasant mood.

Randi calls later, when I am back at Blythedale. I leave Evan and go outside to the parking lot to talk to her. She has just finished having a conference call with Dr Brown, ACS, and Weaver. She had asked Dr Brown if she was sure it was SBS, and Dr Brown had explained at length that she was sure, and that although she was aware there were alternative theories floating around, in this particular case there could be no other diagnosis, not after all the tests that have been performed at Columbia ICU. She is still sure it could only be proven to have happened twice, and not multiple times. That, at least, eases my mind ever so slightly.

Dr Brown also said that, so long as my account of when I left the apartment (at 8am) that day stood up to scrutiny, then there is no possibility I could have inflicted Evan's injuries. They have to have happened very close to the cardiac arrest (which came on at 4.45pm).

After hearing this I start to glaze over, thinking about how Dr Brown has been saying this all along. She never suspected me. So is there anything different about her saying it now? Or will ACS just continue to ignore her?

I am brought back to the conversation when I hear Randi mention something about Norma's account that doesn't sound familiar.

'We all thought that it was unlikely that Norma spent an hour and a half out of the apartment with a baby in a pushchair, even if she did go to Crumbs Bakery for some of that,' she says.

I have never heard that bakery mentioned. Not in Norma's version of events, and not ever, actually. I wonder why not.

When the conversation ends, I come back to Evan's room and pull out my 'Timeline With Exhibits' folder that ACS and Weaver so annoyingly ignored a few weeks ago.

I pick Evan up and sit down with him and my laptop and the file. The ACS case file is a single document, about forty-five pages long, and basically consists of notes typed up by the investigators that visited us at the hospital and by the supervisors. It isn't as difficult to read as I had imagined. I am heartened at least to find two separate entries where the caseworker reports that the NYPD detectives have 'no concern that the mother was the perpetrator'.

I am annoyed to read that the ER doctor reports that when he told me Evan's CT scan was abnormal and that it was SBS, my expression was 'flat', and he thinks that is 'strange'. If he had ever come close to hearing the same kind of thing about his own child, perhaps he would have known better than to judge me in that moment. I am also annoyed to hear that ICU nurse Janene has said that the arching movements I had observed were really only spinal spasms, not actual improvements. I really regret accepting her offer to 'hug it out'.

Eventually, I find the strength to read Norma's account. I don't want to read the report of what happened that afternoon, just like I really don't want to see the video she has taken of Evan's cardiac arrest (which I didn't know about until now). But as I get further into the two paragraphs detailing her account, I am shocked at her statement. It just doesn't have any bearing on what I've always believed to have happened that day.

I pull out the printout of the texts she and I traded on that day and compare them to what she has told ACS.

First, she told Detective Reyes that when Evan initially had breathing issues, in January, she had called 911, but that nobody came. This is completely untrue. She called me and was too panicked to do anything else, so I called 911 from my office. She did not call them at all. We had a full discussion about this afterwards.

As for 17 February, she told ACS that Evan was fussing when she arrived at our apartment that morning. But her text to me, sent about twenty minutes or so after I left, said he was smiling and playing. Then she said that, at lunchtime, he refused to eat anything but a spoonful of cereal. Her text to me at around 1pm said he had eaten all of his cereal.

She told ACS that she had taken Evan out for a walk between 2.30pm and 4pm, during which time she had gone to Crumbs Bakery. But at the hospital she told me she hadn't been out that day. Also, the FDNY emergency response crew had cut off Evan's pyjamas when they arrived (you can see they are the ones he was wearing the night before from the photograph I took of him with the Scottish doll). I don't think it is likely Norma would have taken him out without dressing him first.

I can tell by the dates on the report entries that she was interviewed five days after the cardiac arrest. Apparently enough time to do some research and get her story straight.

I am shocked. I still don't know what happened to Evan, and I still can't be sure of what Norma did, deliberately or otherwise. But one thing has just become crystal clear: she feels the need to lie, and to do so in a fairly elaborate manner. She has to be hiding something.

I think back to my text to her the day after this happened, asking her to give me whatever information she could as it might help the doctors treat Evan. She'd said she had no information. I thought about the many months when the ACS case was focused solely on me, and even now that she has been brought into it, it hasn't taken the pressure off me at all. She knew about it and she knew she had lied to ACS and she stood back — and still stands back — while I go through the court proceeding.

I feel pretty dumb for having been so generous about her in my cover letter to ACS, that's for sure.

13 August 2012

COMPLIANCE CONFERENCE

We have court this morning. Jackie, Deborah and Liz come and sit with me away from the main part of the hallway. We know Norma will be here too and I really do not want to see her. Knowing that she has lied is enough, even without yet knowing what the truth is. The three girls are willing bodyguards.

Randi deals with the attorneys, as usual. I watch, from a distance, as she shows Lubin the three relevant pages of text and the page of the ACS report that shows Norma's inconsistencies, all highlighted in yellow. He practically falls over himself to go and get them photocopied.

When the case is called Randi goes inside the courtroom and asks the judge if my appearance can be excused as I don't want to be in the same room as Norma. Remarkably, the judge says yes.

Twenty minutes or so later, Randi comes out and tells me ACS caseworker Pamela Turner is in the courtroom and has just submitted a letter to the court that the judge has questions about. I am surprised, because I didn't know she was coming, and I haven't seen her in the hallway.

I am more surprised when Randi tells me the judge's questions, though. Turner has written in her report that I refused to consent to Evan going to a long-term care facility, and that I objected to him going to the ICU a few weeks ago. I am furious. She gave me so many assurances when we last met about how this would all be over soon. Then she goes and tells the court a pack of lies.

I am so incensed that I follow Randi right back up the hall, hoping to get into the courtroom to speak to the judge myself. But as we get to the door of the court an overly officious court officer blocks Randi's entrance and tells her that the next case has already been called and she has to submit any corrections in writing. While the two of them are talking, I look into the main part of the hallway. I come eye to eye with Norma. She is sitting alone on one of the waiting-room chairs. Already fired up, I give her a long furious stare. She catches it and then turns her eyes up and to the left, as though this is a natural place for them to sit. Then she looks back again. I am still staring at her. She does the same thing with her eyes again.

My focus on her only stops when Randi and Weaver appear beside me. Weaver turns to Randi first and then to me, saying, 'You may as well hear this, too. My expert hasn't finished her report yet, but she has told me that she strongly believes that only the babysitter can be responsible, given that she was with Evan all day and you weren't.'

I start to cry, big, unattractive, endless sobs. The relief soaks over me. By this point Lubin is standing next to me too, but he obviously already knows the news. Through my tears I ask him if they can let Evan come home with me now, just lift the remand and let us be together in our own apartment.

'I'm sorry,' he says, 'but I have to wait to see what our own expert says first.'

Jackie drives me back to my apartment, where I sit and stare at the walls for several hours, trying to work out what to make of the day.

13 August 2012

A lovely day with Evan. Lots of cuddling and lots of kisses. I have been feeling very calm and connected with him all week – ever since court – it has lifted such a weight off my shoulders. I've only taken one Ativan this week.

After his bath, as I am drying his hair, Evan stares at me full on, with his big blue eyes. Then his jaw starts to move. It lasts a few seconds and then it is gone. It feels like a glimpse of the future.

20 August 2012

Another trip to Scotland, to visit my mum, but another few days without Evan. I sit at the airport bar, feeling my hair go grey. The wine isn't cutting my anxiety one bit. The olives are perhaps the worst I've ever tasted, yet I keep eating them.

I couldn't be better set up for going home. It's only four days and Liz is going to spend two whole days with Evan, and Clare will be there throughout the two days after that. The ACS case is on my mind less and less, and my mum is looking forward to seeing me.

I am very aware that everyone at home will ask me how Evan is, and the truth is that he really isn't any better than the last time I was home. He can wake and sleep now, as opposed to being in a full coma, and he has grown, so he looks very healthy. He even has a couple of teeth. But return of any function has been rare and short-lived.

He will be fine, I know he will – it just takes time. It took my mum ten months to get back to normal after she had her bad turn a few years ago. No one really thought she would get better, but she did. Evan just needs time. And love. I have plenty of both; I just need to stay focused. Seeing him looking at me after his bath a few days ago will carry me for a while.

23 August 2012

GLASGOW, SCOTLAND

I find an old watch of my dad's and put it on. The strap fits perfectly. It reminds me of him whenever I look at it.

I have an appointment with a lady from the Scottish Brain Injury Trust today. I've been looking at my options and think it's a good idea to see what Scotland can offer Evan. I exchanged a few emails with the Trust before I left New York and set up this meeting. As arranged, I sit and wait in the coffee shop of a bookstore on Sauchiehall Street in the centre of Glasgow for half an hour this afternoon. Then I realise I was supposed to meet her yesterday. Aargh! Another example of my inability to think clearly these days. I call, email and text huge apologies. She had been coming from Edinburgh, for goodness sake. She is very kind and doesn't act at all put out.

We Skype when I get back to my mum's house. The lady from

the Trust reminds me that there is a very well-known children's hospital in Glasgow, the Royal Hospital for Sick Children, Yorkhill (it's usually known simply as 'Yorkhill'). It's a 20-minute drive from my mum's house. The lady gives me all sorts of other information about services for children in Scotland with brain injuries, all of which gives me a lot of food for thought.

Angela B and another lifelong friend, Emma, come over in the evening. We sit drinking wine and talking about Evan (I'm not good on any other topic these days). Later, Anne and her partner Richard arrive from England. My mum's front room becomes lively and full of laughter. As we sit chatting, and the wine flows, my mood starts to darken. I remember the stack of old side-plates that are sitting on the counter in the kitchen because my mum wants them thrown out.

Once Angela and Emma leave and Anne and Richard go to bed, I go into the kitchen, and open the back door. It looks out on to a high brick wall, about eight feet away; I am ready for that wall.

One by one, I throw each plate against it.

The plates are not all that satisfying to smash – they give in too easy, and they don't do anything to cut through my increasing anger. So I go back inside and find a can of cream of mushroom soup on the kitchen counter and throw that against the wall. This is a bit better. It makes a satisfying thud as it connects. The tin is still mostly intact, except that it has opened just a tad and some of the cold soup has come out in globs. I retrieve it, planning to do it all over again. I slip on a glob of soup, and find myself down on the ground, amid the splinters of the side plates. My elbow aches. I realise the can of soup has counter-attacked and I decide to consider it a draw and retire.

As I lie in bed, my elbow scraped with dried blood and throbbing, I very much appreciate finally having a physical outlet for my pain. It is being allowed to seep out through the wound, out into the world, at last.

I wake up the next morning feeling quite sore, embarrassed and wondering if I am in any trouble. Anne knocks on my door and brings me in a cup of tea.

'What happened to the plates?' she asks.

'I smashed them against the wall,' I tell her.

'Oh,' she says, and leaves, as though there is nothing unusual about this at all.

I want to go to mass on the Sunday. I know that someone has requested prayers for Evan, and so his name is a constant feature in the weekly bulletin. I want to see it, and perhaps talk to the priest.

Although I genuinely feel comfortable being spiritual rather than religious now, there was a time when I enjoyed going to church too. But then I realised I was gay. With all the insecurities involved in the coming-out process, the Catholic Church seemed only to offer inherent ostracisation to me. I really didn't feel welcome there at all. But I like the Catholic religion, in its pure form. Not judging others is an admirable quality; treating others as you yourself would like to be treated is too.

When John Paul II died I remember feeling quite left out. He had been Pope through my formative years. Even though I feel confident that God made me gay (and that He doesn't make mistakes), I still felt I wasn't welcome at this wake.

Over the years, though, I've realised I had been missing the point. The parts that contradict what I believe in (and of course I'm mostly talking about the homophobia) I can reconcile as the frailty of the humans in the organisation (the Church), and not of the tenets on which it stands. And sometimes, yes, it's those failings that have helped to keep me outside its warm embrace. But, unless it's a direct attack, I have come to realise that Catholicism is no less mine than it is anyone else's. No one has the right to tell me I can't be a Catholic, or that I can't be a good Catholic just because I'm gay. And so I remain as connected to it as I want to be.

As I drink my morning coffee this Sunday, though, I pick up the morning paper and read the front-page news. The main article says that the Scottish Catholic Cardinal has ordered every priest at every mass today to read a prepared letter from the pulpit, telling the congregation that gay marriage, whether religious or civil, is rotting society. I am glad I read that in advance – I don't want to show up somewhere I am not welcome. Still, I can't help thinking it's a shame that I am made to feel like this. It would have been comforting to walk through the Church's doors today.

27 August 2012

BACK IN NEW YORK

Happily back with Evan. We sit and cuddle for hours; I am in my own little heaven. Then the nurse comes in; she says we make a lovely picture. The nicest thing about coming back so refreshed is that I have the energy to soak Evan in fresh love. I think he feels it. At one point he opens his eyes full and wide. He also makes a lot of small movements. And he gives me some great sounds too, especially during his massage.

Dr M comes in next and I ask her about taking him to Scotland. She says it can be done; it will just take a lot of organising. (Then she says she is glad I am back. She sounds like she means it. I feel confused by her once again.)

So, my decision is made: we will aim to move back to Scotland and at the very least see how far we get. I think Evan will do well there. I will do my best.

29 August 2012

Evan looks to very nearly have a grip on his eyes now. They don't roll and loll quite so much.

I make an interesting connection at Yorkhill children's hospital today. I call a number that the Scottish Brain Injury Trust gave me. I am instantly connected to the vent coordinator. She gives me a list of things to do to get the referral in motion. If we can get back there, we can get almost the same home-based services as we would in New York. However, because Glasgow is much smaller than New York, there are less vent-trained carers, and so Evan will be number four on a waiting list. He can stay at Yorkhill while we wait, and they will provide him with excellent care. As much as I would prefer him home with me, it means that Evan and my mum will be in the same city, which will take some strain off me. I can look after both of them without worrying about the other.

In the Cabin tonight a guy tries to buy me a drink. He is a doctor from Westchester Medical Center (and dressed in scrubs). I spare him. In many ways.

31 August 2012

I wake around 5.30am to find two nurses and a doctor standing over Evan.

'What's going on?' I ask.

'He's seizing,' says the nurse.

I look at Evan. I don't think he's seizing. I am very dozy and it takes me a while to get my head together. Then I realise: he isn't seizing, he is breathing. He is taking big goldfish-like gulps of air. He has begun to do this every now and then, but not consistently, and usually when he is in discomfort. I look at his heart rate on the pulse-ox and see that it is elevated, so I ask the doctor to give him a dose of the pain reliever Tylenol. The doctor, meanwhile, is considering giving him a dose of Ativan.

'Don't even think about it,' I caution.

This is exactly why it's so important for me to stay at Evan's bedside. I don't want a repeat of last time. The Tylenol is given and within half an hour of being in my arms he is calm again. Later, I see the tiniest glimpse of white showing along his top gum: another tooth.

I get back to the apartment this evening and manage to speak with the doorman who was on duty the day Evan was taken to hospital. He tells me he is 100 per cent sure that Evan and Norma did not go out that afternoon. He came on at 3pm and the only time he saw them was when the ambulance was wheeling Evan out.

'I just remember seeing his lifeless little body on the stretcher,' he adds.

I could have done without hearing that.

3 September 2012

LABOUR DAY

Today is Evan's first birthday. It is also Labour Day in the US, which is significant because it's a holiday and it means the hospital is nice and quiet, so the day is pleasantly low-key. Sure enough, this morning I can't help but let quite a few tears escape. These tears are for me, though – Evan is doing fine. I just feel so sorry for myself. It is the anniversary of the happiest day of my life, and I miss my baby boy so much. I don't let myself go there often any more, but I can't hold it in today.

Violet, his godmother, is in town from Ireland for the weekend to share Evan's birthday with us. Friends asked if I wanted to throw a party for him and invite people. I knew far better than to plan something like that, after the sob-fest that was his six-month birthday. So I made dinner and lunch plans with some of them over the weekend so I could see them, but I kept today quite free. Except for Violet. She is the perfect person to spend it with. She shows up today with a couple of very delicious looking cakes and a ton of presents from her and from other friends in Ireland. We dress Evan in some of his new birthday clothes and we sing a few songs to him. I know a few more tears are on their way, but I also know that I don't need to try and hide them from Violet.

6 September 2012

SW2 says that representatives from a long-term care place in Wanaque, New Jersey, are going to be coming to see us today.

'Don't worry,' she assures me, 'They are meeting with every vent child.'

She explains that although they do now have a couple of new vent beds available, they won't take Evan as there are several babies ahead of him at Blythedale. She tells me to humour them. 'Just go through the motions,' she says. 'Put on a show.'

'Oh, I'll put on a show, alright,' I reply.

She looks worried.

When they arrive, I ask them about therapies and what – and how often – Evan will receive them if he goes to Wanaque.

'We all sit down and discuss Evan's needs and come up with a therapy plan to suit,' one offers.

'I've heard that before,' I tell them, 'and it never seems to work out in our favour.'

'Well… it depends,' she offers, with a polite smile.

'Yes, I've heard that before too,' I reply, not smiling.

I explain to them that we really don't want to go to Wanaque. I tell them how important it is to me to sleep every night beside Evan's bed, and that I know this is not an option at Wanaque. I also explain that I hope to regain custody after the trial mid-November, and that it seems futile to move him to their long-term care facility if he is only going to move again, to Scotland, shortly after. They leave, and I feel that I have made my point well.

7 September 2012

SW2 visits today to tell me that she has asked ACS if they object to Blythedale writing a referral for Evan for the Scottish hospital. ACS has responded, saying they will not oppose it. That's very big of them, I tell her. There's no moving them on the immediate issue, of course: the fact that the state technically has custody over Evan, and for no good reason.

I meet Liz in Valhalla for dinner. We have fried clams and beer and I vent almost the entire time. Afterwards I wait for her to catch her train back to the city. Her ears must be ringing all the way back to Brooklyn. I power myself all the way up the hill home, in the dark, still obsessing.

11 September 2012

I wake up to Evan singing. I can't think of a better way to start the day. Of course, he is only phonating – his tongue and mouth still don't work – but it is beautiful, nonetheless.

The air is clear and clean now that it's a bit cooler, and the autumn leaves are starting to make their mark. I went back to the city yesterday for another short break. Standing on a subway platform to take a train to my apartment, I receive an email from SW2. It says that Wanaque have made a formal offer of a vent bed for Evan.

I am stunned. Once again I can feel our entire world shifting.

SW2 ends the email by asking if I want to appeal the decision. Under the rules (whose rules, I really don't know) you can file an appeal the day before the scheduled transfer and, within 72 hours, you get an answer.

It seems there is a very good chance this move will happen, even if I do appeal. It's not as dire a prospect as it once felt; the ACS case seems to have turned a corner in my favour and hopefully Evan and I can go to Scotland in a few months anyway. Besides, change can sometimes be good, and perhaps we need a bit of a change. Then again, with change comes turmoil too. And sometimes it's better to stick with the devil you know. I tell her yes, I will appeal. At least this gives me a few more days to adjust.

As planned, I meet a friend for a glass of wine at the Loeb Boathouse in Central Park. I try to explain the situation in rational terms to her, without showing the shock and fear I am feeling. This turns out to be a good exercise because it helps me to think clearly about it, without panicking.

After that, I go over to my cousin Madeleine's house. She has just moved to New York from Vancouver and is working at the United Nations (both she and her husband Dave are attorneys too). Incredibly she found an apartment right around the corner from ours (without knowing where we live). I've only met her a couple of times before but Schwarz cousins (and there are more than thirty of us) have an unwritten code of instant friendship with each other.

Madeleine and Dave's two boys, aged nine and six, provide much-needed light entertainment for the first part of the evening, and once they go to bed, a couple of bottles of wine between us provides even lighter entertainment for the second half. This was until Madeleine asks what had happened to Evan. I don't know if it is the wine, the comfort level of being with family, or just a longing to share for a bit, but I eventually spill the entire story out to them: the babysitter, the first hospitalisation, the ACS case, everything. They are, of course, both lovely and extremely sympathetic, but practical too, and ask if I need any help. Just talking about it is help enough for now, I tell them.

This morning I wake up around 10.30am, feeling the wine from last night and, as usual, missing Evan terribly. Still in bed, I check my messages and find one from Randi. She has forwarded me an email from the Weaver lawyer, and includes Weaver's expert's report. In the expert's professional opinion, it says, as I had been out since 8am and Evan had gone into cardiac arrest after 4pm, there is no way I could have had anything to do with what happened to him.

This is a huge breakthrough, of course, but also bittersweet – the report goes into much greater detail about Evan's injuries than I am ready for. There is a little light humour to be had, I suppose, in the fact that the doctor who wrote the report is actually called Dr Kathryn Grimm.

Coincidentally, the expert Randi hired also delivers his

findings to her later today. He has the same conclusion – that it could not possibly have been me – but based on a slightly different theory, along with some additional details that Dr Grimm has not considered. (Like I say, doctors often differ in their opinions.)

I get the train from Grand Central to White Plains and, just as it has come out of the tunnel and is passing through Harlem, I check my emails again. This time there is one from SW2. She writes that there is good news waiting for me at the hospital, and that I am probably ready for some.

I don't want to hope too much.

'If it's that Andy Murray won the US Open last night, I already know,' I reply.

'No, it's that ACS called to say they are withdrawing the petition against you and seeking to have the remand removed,' is the reply.

'Thank you for making me cry on a crowded train,' I write back.

The train can't get to Westchester fast enough. When I eventually get back to Blythedale, I stride in like I have just bought the place. I pick Evan up and sit cuddling him, laughing and crying all at the same time. Quite a few people come in to congratulate me, and I tell anyone and everyone I happen to meet in the corridors, 'We're going home.' Everyone is very pleased for us; it is wonderful.

The ACS case against me can't continue. I will no longer have to fight against the move to Wanaque. After six months of being treated like an unfit mother it is almost too much to take in.

Half an hour after I get back, Dr M and SW2 come in to talk about us going home. Paulina the discharge nurse arrives too. I know she doesn't have the most appealing title, but she is in charge of organising patients' release home. I've seen her so many times, when each one of our room-mates has been well enough to leave us behind and go home. I have been fantasising about the day she walks in to see us: this day.

Paulina takes some details from me and tells me she will set things in motion for going home. I call my mum once she and Dr M leave. I really want to share the good news with her, but, of course, we have all protected her from the ACS issue. So I start the conversation with, 'Do you want the good news or the bad news first?'

'The bad news,' she says, as I knew she would.

'Well, there's no bad news so you'll have to have the good news.'

'Okay then!'

'Evan and I are moving back to Scotland.'

She is delighted, although very surprised, as I haven't mentioned it to her before in case it wasn't possible.

'I was just thinking today about how much I hate living alone,' she says.

She is so happy that she makes me promise to tell her all over again tomorrow.

12 September 2012

The euphoria continues today. We get word that I have to go to court tomorrow to watch Lubin eat humble pie when he requests the judge allow ACS to withdraw the case against me.

13 September 2012

I meet Randi and Liz outside the courtroom after a mad dash downtown due to unusually bad subway traffic. Jackie and Deborah join us there, both looking flustered at having been stuck in traffic, too.

'I am not missing this!' exclaims Jackie as she runs up and hugs me.

Norma is here too, sitting a few rows away from us, with her mother and her lawyer. I don't look at her this time, but I do look at her mother. I want to convey in that look that she and I are both mothers, that's all.

I watch Norma later, though, walking down the hall to the restroom and in the courtroom. She doesn't look like someone who is worried, not about herself and not about a poor little boy still on a life-support machine and terribly injured. Instead she looks confident and calm – and, I feel, somewhat detached from the proceedings. Maybe she is just covering her nerves.

The girls sit behind us as Randi and I, and Norma and her lawyer take to the tables and, along with ACS and Weaver, we all stand as the judge enters. He listens to ACS ask for the petition to be withdrawn against me, and he listens to Norma's lawyer argue that it still doesn't mean I didn't hurt Evan, just that I didn't hurt him that day.

The judge is dismissive of this argument but then he goes on a rant against Lubin about how the expert report goes too far. He says Dr Grimm has given a conclusion of law in stating that Norma was the perpetrator, when she was only allowed to give a statement of opinion. That really seems to be splitting hairs, given that Shaken Baby Syndrome, when diagnosed by doctors, is actually a legal diagnosis, which is a conclusion of law. I am not about to argue the theoretical merits of the distinction, though.

Both Lubin and Weaver look suitably cowed (but then they always do in front of this judge). The judge goes on about it for so long that I start to think he is going to deny the application to get me out of the case. Eventually though, he gets to the word that lawyers always yearn for in a situation like this: 'However...' And then he explains why he is dismissing the case against me despite his reservations about the expert report.

While this probably doesn't feel so great for Lubin and Weaver, the judge is actually doing them both a huge favour: he is putting them to the sword. He is signalling to them that if they show up at Norma's trial with nothing but that report he will give them a really hard time over it. He is handing them the opportunity to improve on it.

The judge then turns to Norma's lawyer and reminds him to direct his client to come back for her trial on 15 November.

Norma leaves the courtroom immediately, and we slowly start to pack up so as to avoid bumping into her in the hallway.

Then the officious court officer comes over and tells us to clear out, the next case is waiting to be heard.

I walk over to Lubin, who is putting his folder in his briefcase, avoiding his lunch box. I extend a hand, and when he takes it I tell him, 'I can't thank you, because of what you put me through, but I do ask that you pursue the babysitter properly, to find out the truth, for my sake and for Evan's sake.'

He stares at me for a moment, then turns away.

When we get outside, Lubin comes over to me, unbidden this time, while Randi is talking to the girls.

'I don't mean to be cruel,' he starts (oh, here we go), 'but the decision to withdraw the case against you was 110 per cent out of my hands. It went all the way to the Commissioner. And the decision to withdraw against the babysitter would be out of my hands too, if that's what happens.'

He really is just being mean: he has just been beaten down by an angry judge and then he's had me in his face, rubbing things in. And he is young. But I am in no mood to give him any leeway.

'The hell you put me through, during the worst time of my life, what my family went through, and what these friends went through, they all had to watch me suffer. The emotional toll and then the financial toll... And now you've got actual evidence against the babysitter and you've got all the extra help I've already given you and you think there's a chance you might drop the case against her?'

By the looks of him he realises he has gone too far, and also that he isn't enjoying being the focus of another one of my tirades.

Afterwards, Randi, the girls and I go for a coffee and sit in tears and laughter, going over the day, point after point, blow by blow.

14 September 2012

A nice man stops by my apartment this morning to check the sockets to make sure they are safe for Evan's vent when he comes home.

On my way back to Grand Central I go to Tiffany's and buy two teacups. Then I pick up some nice boxes of tea and take the package to Randi's office. She is delighted to see me, and when she sees the coral Tiffany bag she says, 'Oh, you didn't!' That's the problem with the Tiffany shopping bag – it looks like what's inside must be worth more than two teacups and some tea bags actually cost. She seems touched nonetheless.

And then off I go, back, once again, to Grand Central, to take the train to see my beautiful boy.

When I get back to the hospital I see two of the mothers I had meditated with. 'We're going home,' I blurt out, and then immediately wish I hadn't. They are both a long way off that, even though their children are showing more progress than Evan. Nevertheless, they look very pleased for us.

16 September 2012

My friend Brian shows up this morning and takes me for breakfast. I tell him everything that's happened with the ACS case. It is so much easier to talk about it now it's over. We celebrate with a roll and scrambled egg and ham from the deli.

Later, I am trained in how to use the portable vent at home. I already know a lot about the vent, but being taught how it works gives me much more confidence. I get shown how to handle it when we go outside. It's relatively straightforward, but you have to be okay with looking like an astronaut with all the battery packs, suction equipment and other things hanging off your back, shoulders and arms. Very portable, I'm sure.

I know we are only in the seventh month, but it feels like the worst part was the first six months. They were dark, and now they are over: there is more light now.

24 September 2012

I am furious all over again: Pamela Turncoat has called me offering 'services' for Evan. I tell her to go away and not to bother us any more. The ACS case is over and Evan is entirely in my care, not hers. She tells me they still have supervision over Evan. I am livid.

I get Randi to write a letter to ACS, telling them to send me written instructions as to what my obligations are now that the case against me has been dropped.

25 September 2012

I was so riled up last night after the ACS issue that I took an Ativan to try and get to sleep. I've been groggy all day as a result. More side effects from ACS — will it ever stop? Evan was quite out of sorts today too. He postured a lot.

27 September 2012

Depression follows me. After the excitement of the past couple of weeks and the elation it brought, I've started to feel low, so low. I walk through Central Park. It's a beautiful sunny day, but I keep seeing families and mothers and infants and toddlers, and it makes me feel so sad. All these ordinary, normal lives. My life is not normal, I don't fit in here right now. I come home and crawl into bed in the middle of the afternoon and stay there for a good few hours.

Ironically, it seems the anxiety around the ACS case at least distracted me from a lot of the reality of Evan's condition. Now that it's over, and I don't have to worry about it any more, I am back to focusing entirely on what the new normal is for Evan and me. The adjustment has stalled over the last few months, but now I have to face it full on.

The worst thing about feeling down is that I stop feeling positive about Evan and then I feel guilty, like I'm losing faith in our future. I have to keep reminding myself that I must send Evan positive energy as much and as often as I can. It's not easy, and it's not even all that natural: hope and acceptance don't necessarily make good bedfellows to each other. But hope is full of positive energy and it's a lot lighter to carry than negative energy.

Blythedale

29 September 2012

Pamela Turncoat shows up at the hospital today. SW2 comes in with her, looking apologetic again. We chat for a bit. I am very mature, all things considered (the circumstances, not the fact that I am forty-one). The funny thing about Pamela is that she is actually very likeable, when she's not wrecking your life. She has a lively nature, and is quick to smile. She notices Evan has his eyes open and is moving them about (ever so slightly – I think it was more because I was moving him, to be honest) – and she gets quite excited about this. She is very friendly and positive, and I start to suspect that maybe she is in the right profession after all. Very few people in her position could have walked into our room and held a conversation with me after all that has come to pass.

Drama!

As I change Evan's trach ties this evening he has a spasm and arches up, and his trach comes right out. I can't get it back in and he can't get any air and starts turning purple. I call for the nurse but can't see her in the pod and so I hit the code blue button. As usual, within seconds the room is full and, also as usual, thank God, the problem is solved immediately. One of the nurses asks me if I want to sit down; I don't.

'Are you sure?' she asks kindly, 'I was here the last time this happened and you needed to sit down then.'

But I really am fine this time – I have managed to break through the wall of fear. Although I haven't fixed the problem myself, I have remained calm and in control.

Strength is a muscle: the more you work it, the more you have.

3O September 2O12

I meet with a lawyer with a good reputation for taking cases against ACS today. We chat for over an hour. In the end he agrees to look over the medical records.

'I wasn't sure if you had a case when we talked on the phone,' he offers, 'but having met with you and listened to what happened, I think you might.'

Whether or not I can sue ACS is kind of irrelevant at this stage. Right now I just need to be sure to pursue every avenue, so that I don't wake up ten years from now and wonder why I didn't react.

8 October 2O12

There's been a lot of activity in these last few weeks. The plan now is that Evan and I go home to our apartment in Manhattan as soon as we can. Then after two weeks, so long as he has remained stable on his portable vent the entire time, I can take him on a plane to Glasgow, where he will go straight to Yorkhill Children's Hospital, until such time as we can get home care to allow him to come home. I will move back in with my mum and spend my days with Evan at the hospital.

In preparation for bringing Evan to Scotland, I spent last weekend in Glasgow, to check out the facilities available for him. Anne came to New York and babysat Evan, and Pauline came to Glasgow to visit Yorkhill with me.

We took a tour of the hospital and met a few of the nurses and administrators, including the 'ventilation support coordinator'. It was very helpful having Pauline there. She was supportive but also took notes and asked questions. The vent coordinator was very practical but didn't express so much as a hint of negativity about Evan's condition or prognosis. I had been worried something would be said to make me break down in tears, but it wasn't like that at all– it just all felt positive and accepting.

The hospital is big and has its own ICU unit, so if Evan becomes sick while he is there he will simply go to a different floor, not a different hospital. The wards are a little bigger and are open-plan, so there is more activity going on and, therefore, more stimulation for the children.

Parents can spend as much time as they want there, but they can't stay the night as there is no bed for them. So long as I can spend as much time as possible with Evan all day long, I'm quite pleased to have no option but to go home and sleep in a proper bed every night.

There are beautiful Scottish views from the ward windows. The River Clyde is on one side, wind farms in the distance on another, and beautiful Scottish mountains on the third. The hospital is not as new or as stunning as Blythedale, but it's very clean and there seems to be a lot more stimulation as the beds are not isolated into pods as they are in Blythedale. There are similar services available in terms of therapies and home-care nursing. I really can't think of any reason not to come.

I Believe in Evan

We had wonderful sunshine all weekend long, and the autumn leaves were beautiful. I had to resist the allure of the weather, though. It's a fickle friend all right. No one goes to Scotland for the climate.

10 October 2012

I have Evan dressed in the new red corduroy trousers, blue Oxford shirt and knitted vest I brought him back from Glasgow. He looks very handsome and staff keep coming in to check him out. I used to work with a chef who came into work in a suit one day (as opposed to chef whites). He said he was feeling poorly so he got dressed up in his best clothes to feel better. I just remembered that recently. Given all the oohs and aahs Evan is getting today, I realise what good advice that is.

17 October 2012

I have a meeting with the therapists at Blythedale's equipment clinic. They show me a pushchair and a bath that I can get through Evan's health insurance. It is overwhelming seeing all this heavy-duty equipment for my wee boy. I'm stepping into a new world, one that I never contemplated. It's not easy but I guess you just have to run with it. What other options are there?

We have a different nurse today, a new one. We start chatting and after a while she looks at Evan and says, 'Don't ever underestimate a child. I've seen cases where I think, dear

God, and then they go on and make a full recovery. Don't ever lose faith.'

I won't.

23 October 2012

Today is the first anniversary of my dad's death. Coincidentally, it is also the fourteenth anniversary of Connie Connolly's death. I wonder if she's giving his shoes a special polish in heaven right now like she used to do every morning before he went to work (brown brush on, red brush off).

I call Detective Reyes. I haven't heard anything at all from her since she called Jackie after ACS first brought charges against me. It turns out she got promoted and has moved on to another office. Sergeant Accomando has taken over the case. I speak with him and tell him I am concerned that I haven't heard anything at all from ACS or the NYPD.

'I just need to know what happened to Evan,' I tell him. 'And I'm worried the opportunity to find out will be wasted.'

Sergeant Accomando reads the notes to me. Lubin has actually logged every single point I had sent him into the computer file on the case. He had added, 'It would be a gross injustice if the babysitter is not investigated further in this matter.'

Okay, so at least he has done what he should have done as far as the NYPD go. But would it have been going too far for Lubin to let the mother (me) know that he had relayed this to the NYPD?

Sergeant Accomando tells me there will be a status meeting

with ACS, Dr Brown, and the District Attorney in a few weeks, and that he will get back to me.

26 October 2012

For the second time in ten days Evan has shown signs of teariness. His face still can't move at all (except for the slow and semi-closing eyelids, but his eyelids get red up to the brow and tears fall from the sides of his eyes). His physical therapist handed him back to me today because she could see how upset he looked. I was so happy to take him. After a while, the redness went away. What a lovely feeling to know that your child's unhappiness can be cured by your holding him: my gift to Evan, and his to me.

We are still waiting to hear when we will get nurses for home care – we can't be discharged until they are in place. I can't believe it's taking so long.

3 November 2012

HURRICANE SANDY

Last year Hurricane Irene came to town the weekend before I had Evan. It was an exciting time. In the hours before she hit, every store had a queue out the door and items disappeared fast as everyone tried to grab enough supplies to see them through. I stocked up like everyone else, but, being 38 weeks pregnant, most of my stash was eaten an hour or so before the storm was due to hit.

Mayor Bloomberg ordered a shutdown of the city and the streets were empty. The storm came and went overnight, but was far weaker than expected. Although it caused quite extensive damage upstate and on Long Island, it did almost nothing to New York City. We all laughed at our own overreactions.

A few days ago we were warned to expect 'Hurricane Sandy'. People in coastal towns in New Jersey and parts of Queens and Brooklyn, as well as on Long Island and other parts of New York, were told to evacuate. Many assumed it would be just like Irene and no big deal and so they didn't leave their homes and businesses.

The storm hit on Monday evening and kept going through Tuesday morning. I stayed at the hospital as I would have done anyway, although I had no real choice since all transportation had been shut down the day before. All of the hospital staff on duty on the Monday day shift stayed overnight and slept in various rooms and workspaces. The hospital provided free breakfast, dinner and lunch for two days.

It really is a good thing that Evan and I are still at Blythedale. If we had been at home, even though our neighbourhood wasn't one of the worst hit, we would have had the constant worry that the electricity would go out. Also, the home-care nurses probably wouldn't have been able to get to us. I would have had to remain awake twenty-four hours a day, every day just to make sure Evan was okay.

Blythedale had two new generators installed as part of its refurbishment last year. They cost $2.5 million to install and are contained underground. The day before the storm they had fired up the first one, and it had worked so effectively, they didn't even need to use the second one, which was only there as back up. As a result, we didn't have any problems at Blythedale at all. I saw the lights in our room flicker twice, but other than that I didn't notice anything. I couldn't even hear the wind against the windows in our room, and I sleep an inch away from them.

Other places weren't as lucky. New York University Langone Hospital on the east side of downtown Manhattan bore the brunt of things when the East River burst its banks. That hospital had tested its generators the week before the storm, but no one had realised the water surges and the rain would be so heavy. Their electrical units were in the basement, which was very quickly flooded and everything shorted. The generators should have been able to take over, but they were on the roof and quickly became flooded and unworkable too. More than 200 patients had to be evacuated, including many newborn babies on vents. Because their vents were not the portable kind, they had to be carried down fifteen flights of stairs, all the time being ambued by hospital staff. It gives me chills to think how terrifying that must have been.

Outside our hospital, for as far as you could see, there was no power at all. Trees had fallen on electrical wires, and power outages occurred due to flooding and fires. Not so much further away, in the city and in the coastal towns, dozens of people had been killed. Towns had been washed away and block after block of housing had burned down.

All of Lower Manhattan was flooded and plunged into darkness. Everything was shut down. TV reports showed footage of well-dressed people rummaging through supermarket dumpsters to try and get food.

On Staten Island, a mother had been driving her SUV home, trying to get her two- and four-year-old sons to safety. A surge of water surrounded her car and stalled it. She got the boys out of the car and held them tight. Another surge came and both boys were swept from her arms. Their bodies were found two days later.

There is always someone worse off.

7 November 2012

Evan opened and closed his eyes so much today, and made some hand movements. Massaging his right shoulder made his left hand do a lot. I love him so much. I think he has just had a big improvement – he definitely lets you know when he's happy or not, by the way he phonates. He makes a sort of purring sound. I love it.

Because of Hurricane Sandy, the hospital decided to postpone Halloween until today so the children in the hospital and the school could hold their annual parade. I dressed Evan up in a lion's outfit – he looked very fierce and brave.

8 November 2012

Lubin has not contacted me and there is only one week to go before Norma's trial in the Family Court case. He hasn't subpoenaed me as a witness and he hasn't asked me for any information. I'm worried that he is going to screw it all up and I will never know what happened to Evan.

And no one has responded to Randi's last letter. I still don't know what 'supervision of Evan' means or what I'm supposed to do to comply. What if I'm already not complying? Will they bring another action against me?

I emailed Sergeant Accomando a few days ago. He replied that they still hadn't done much work on the case and blamed the hurricane (which put most of Manhattan out of service for two weeks, so I couldn't really argue with him).

15 November 2012

NORMA'S TRIAL DATE

I slept in my own bed till noon yesterday, and then had lunch in Midtown with my friend Barbara. When she went back to work I came home and climbed right back in to bed.

I wake up with a few hours to spare this morning. I put on my suit and take the subway downtown. I arrive in the courthouse in plenty of time this time around. Randi isn't here – there is no need. Pamela Turner is, though, and is her usual cheery self. Lubin walks past us but doesn't acknowledge either of us. This makes Pamela laugh, her usual easy laugh. 'He thinks he's all that and then some,' I say, smiling. She laughs some more.

Weaver shows up early too, for once, and joins us. As the three of us talk, Norma, her sister and her lawyer walk by.

Norma sees me but keeps walking. She looks relaxed. I feel a surge of raw emotion. I tell Weaver I can feel myself starting to lose control a bit at the sight of her, so she, Weaver, walks me over to the elevators, out of sight of Norma, to explain today's court process to me.

She tells me she believes Norma is going to submit to the court's jurisdiction and accept a finding of child abuse against her. This is kind of like pleading the Fifth Amendment. She isn't going to testify and incriminate herself in this piddling family court case because, although the sanctions aren't huge (some counselling and a twenty-eight-year ban on working with children), her testimony might be used against her in a criminal case.

On the one hand, I'm glad I won't have to hear testimony from experts and doctors describing Evan's condition. On the other, though, I have really wanted to hear what Norma has to say for herself. Submitting to the court's jurisdiction means she won't testify at all (not until the criminal case, whenever that is). I feel robbed but I also feel relieved.

Lubin is milling around at this point, and can see me trying to catch his eye, so he chooses this moment to have a long chat with the officious court officer. Eventually the officer manages to pry himself away and Lubin has no choice but to talk to me.

'What is going on with the criminal case?' I ask him.

'In terms of what?'

'Are they going to arrest her?'

'My understanding is that there will probably be charges brought in a few months.'

By the looks of things it almost kills him to divulge this to me, in case it might actually be of benefit to me to know it. Still, it is more than I have heard from Sergeant Accomando.

The court officer steps into the hallway, 'Parties on Leonce!' he calls.

We all file in. This time around I have to sit in one of the two rows available for members of the public. I sit behind the ACS and Weaver side, rather than behind Norma's. I know full well that my mood is combustible, and that I am doing us all a favour by keeping as far away from her as possible. I even make sure there are bodies in the way so I can't see her easily. A handful of attorneys sit around me, waiting for cases after this one.

The proceedings get underway. At the judge's invitation, Norma's lawyer stands up and tells the court that his client is indeed willing to submit to the court's jurisdiction and accept a finding of child abuse against her. After some discussion, the judge rules that in addition to having her name entered on the Central Registry as a child abuser, she cannot work with children for the next twenty-eight years, she cannot have any contact with Evan until his eighteenth birthday, and she will be placed under ACS's supervision for the next three months, during which time she will have to attend parenting classes and undergo a mental evaluation.

The judge invites input from both ACS and Weaver. Lubin stands up and tells the judge a criminal case is pending. I look at Norma and she doesn't flinch at this. As a matter of fact, the only time I see any trace of emotion is at one point when the judge is explaining something to her and she smiles in accord. Given that she is in the process of being labelled a child abuser, she is remarkably sanguine.

The lawyers each stand at the appropriate times and do their talking. No longer a defendant, I can get a better view of each of them in their respective roles. All three are cautious and lacking in confidence when they speak in court. Maybe it is just this judge – he is certainly cranky – but even so, a lawyer can't afford to do anything but exude as much confidence as possible in a courtroom. If you don't feel confident, you have to fake it till you make it. You absolutely owe it to your client to show your very best side.

This judge, as far as I can tell, can smell their fear and is intent on punishing each of them for it at every opportunity.

Weaver stands up and asks for the medical records to be entered into evidence. The judge doesn't even wait for Norma's lawyer to object (and he may have no objection at all) and denies her request. 'You should have stipulated to that before you came in here,' he says, angrily. This is petty of him and is not at all designed to help Evan, I feel. I throw up my hands in dramatic protest.

'What is that, at the back?' he shouts, angrily, at me.

'That's my son you're talking about,' I reply, without any of the fear of the three attorneys.

'And?'

(Oh good, he is taking me on, inviting me to speak.)

'And I'm more interested in having Ms Leonce explain to the court exactly what she did to my son.'

The female attorneys beside me stop their chattering, and the male attorney at the other end of the bench puts down his paper (which he has been irritatingly rustling throughout the hearing). I am ready to take everyone on but the judge very calmly picks up his pen and starts writing on his notepad. I have no idea what he is writing. Possibly something along the lines of, 'Uh oh, that crazy Scottish woman is getting fired up again. If I don't catch her eye she might stop.' Whatever it was though, he writes for so long that it gives both of us enough time to let calm heads prevail once again. When he is done, he looks up and starts asking entirely unrelated questions of Lubin.

Lubin then hands the judge a 'status update' for Evan, written on Blythedale letterhead, which is always submitted on court days. Another good thing about no longer appearing in court as a party – and therefore without an attorney – is that I am not privy to the contents of these letters. I don't have to suffer seeing the black and white type of 'there has been no significant improvement' written by someone who doesn't sit and hold Evan, and her hopes, in her arms all day, every day.

'What's the hold up with the release from Blythedale?' the judge asks both Weaver and Lubin.

Neither has any idea and both sit gormlessly looking at their files. I raise my hand.

'Okay,' he says, apparently willing to take the risk of letting me speak again.

I am feeling better at this stage and stand and explain that the nursing-care package has not yet been finalised. Then he asks about the 'therapy' package that ACS say it is trying to arrange for me. Pamela Turner answers these questions and explains it will take about three months to start.

'Has it been explained to you why it will take three months, Ms Schwarz?'

I don't want to get caught up in a discussion about what ACS can do. I also don't want to discuss our move to Scotland, not in front of ACS and Norma – it's not their business.

'It just takes time, Your Honour,' I tell him.

'Yes, well these things do take time and we get used to them taking time, but it doesn't mean we have to put up with it,' he says, smiling over his glasses at me.

'Your Honour, given everything I do put up with these days, with respect, that's a very minor issue.'

He has already looked down and doesn't look back up again. Wisely.

He removes the order of 'supervision' over Evan (whatever that was) and closes the case. The courtroom begins to empty. I deliberately hang back, knowing better than to leave at the same time as Norma. My last ten years of working in court have at least taught me a certain amount of discipline, and I know there is a limit to the level of outburst the court will put up with. But I have no idea what I will do if I am face to face with Norma, and I really don't fancy my chances of staying calm around her.

Lubin turns to me: 'Come on, we have to get out.'

'I'm not putting myself in her vicinity,' I explain calmly.

A female court officer comes over to where we are now standing.

'You have to leave, the next case is coming in.'

'I promise you, if you put me in a position where I am close to that woman, I will physically attack her.'

I am surprised to hear myself say this. And I am also surprised to hear the court officer say, 'I understand.' Then she continues, 'There is an entryway you can stand in until she leaves and I'll make sure you don't get near her.'

So that's what we do.

Pamela Turner stands in the hallway talking to Norma, getting her details so she can supervise her over the next few months. The court officer stands on the corridor side of the courtroom door, and I stand in the entryway, with Lubin, staring at Norma.

'I'll walk you to the lift if you want,' he says.

I don't fancy Jesse Lubin's chances of protecting me from my own emotions, so I opt to stay where I am, inside the little vestibule. The officer stands watch until Norma gets into the elevator and then stands aside so I can leave too. I am more than a little grateful to her for doing this.

Just before Lubin and I leave our stakeout spot I say to him, 'This probably won't come as a surprise to you, but I've just retained a lawyer to sue ACS on my behalf.'

I can see him starting to object.

'I know you're not a decision-maker, and I'm not even asking for your opinion, but I'm giving you the opportunity to go to your supervisor or whoever it is you should go to and explain that and ask if they want to settle now. I have spent $20,000 on legal fees defending myself. But if they're going to settle with me, they have to do it now or they lose that opportunity.'

I have no idea whether I have a case against ACS, but I do know that this is my one and only opportunity to give Lubin a metaphorical knee in the gut before we part ways.

'Thanks for the heads-up,' he says, and turns on his heel, pushing the door and walking out into the hallway.

I ask Pamela what the conversation with Norma was like. She tells me she reminded her that the finding of child abuse will remain in place for twenty-eight years and that there will be a criminal case too, so not to go anywhere. I ask her how Norma reacted.

'She just said, "I will pray."'

This catches me a little off guard.

Later, I am surprised at how visceral my reaction to Norma was. I really thought I had reconciled her role in this and had forgiven her. And yet I had an instinctively strong reaction against her.

As a matter of fact, I find myself often praying about Norma. I pray that she was negligent and stupid but that she didn't hurt Evan out of badness. I pray that it didn't happen more than the two times Dr Brown can confirm. I pray that Norma can live with herself, and that she doesn't commit suicide under the weight of guilt that she may be feeling. I do not want that. I pray that the justice system does what it has to do fairly, and with little or no input from me.

I pray for myself too. I pray that I don't allow anger to consume me. That I can stay positive for Evan. That I can keep forgiving Norma when I do find out what she did.

More than anything, of course, I pray for Evan. I pray that he improves and that this all becomes a thing of the past, not a lifelong sentence for him.

I wish too. I wish that none of this had happened. I wish that Evan and I are battling his teething together; that we are laughing as he throws his toys around; that I put him to bed only for him to call for me to read another story. I wish I could hear him laugh. I wish I could hear him cry.

Later, I email everyone who knew about the ACS case (and that's still only about ten people in total) and tell them what has happened in brief terms. I tell them I really don't want to talk about this aspect any more.

17 November 2012

I've spent the last two days with Evan as he nurses a cold. His nose runs and his heart rate is low because he's wiped out. He has to get suctioned more often because he has catarrh in his chest and can't cough it up. As for me, well, I don't want to talk to anyone. I don't want to think. I should possibly feel relief that the ACS case is over, but I don't – I just feel immense sadness.

We're a right pair right now.

19 November 2012

Dr M has sent us for an X-ray to see whether Evan's cold has led to a chest infection. Nurse Nancy unhooks Evan from the wall sockets and together we roll him (in his buggy) all the way down the hall, past the cafeteria, to the X-ray room in the old part of the building where the outpatient hospital is.

I feel oddly self-conscious. I don't think Evan has left that room since we were in the ICU in August. We pass by a load of different people, all of them looking at Evan in his big oversized buggy.

I remember taking my mum out shopping in her wheelchair when it first became too tiring for her to walk long distances. After a few times she started saying she didn't want to go out any more. With much probing she told me the problem was the wheelchair: she couldn't stand the way people looked at her when she was in it. She said it made her feel like less of a person.

This being a hospital full of sick children, of course people aren't looking at Evan like he is an unusual looking child. Everyone here is unusual looking when compared to able-bodied children. Instead, though, I am aware that they are taking a look at Evan to see how cute he is, like people used to do when I took him for a walk in the park. They don't seem to be focused on the disability or the vent or the wheelchair at all. But I still feel very self-conscious.

I guess the problem right now is me.

I've started to realise that I'm feeling anxious about taking Evan home. I've been telling the people in our apartment building that he is getting better and better and that he will eventually be fine. It's not that that's not true, I believe it. But I'm aware that I've been telling them what I think it is that they want to hear, and they might not be prepared for the scale of Evan's condition. And that worries me. I don't want sympathy and I don't want tears but I also don't want shock. I want everyone to see the beauty in my lion-hearted boy, and nothing else.

I'm aware I may be asking too much.

22 November 2012

THANKSGIVING

It's a beautiful late autumn day. The sun is out and the air is crisp. Hurricane Sandy left just enough brown leaves on the trees to create a Thanksgiving feeling.

The hospital posted signs earlier this week to say there will be a Thanksgiving dinner in the cafeteria for everyone today. I sit around waiting for someone to come and take us there. No one does though, and it's getting late, so eventually I ask our nurse what the plan is. She is Nepalese and not long in the USA so she isn't very invested in the holiday. She asks Madison, who is on duty on the other half of our pod, and comes back with the message, 'It's only for the big kids – Evan can't eat so there's no point.'

I like the Nepalese nurse and I know she isn't trying to be mean, but that stings. I walk down to the cafeteria to get some food to take back to the room. There are all kinds of families and children there, as well as lots of staff members. It's a jovial atmosphere.

'Screw this,' I think.

I go back to our room, get our nurse to help unhook Evan and get him ready for the road, and then wheel him down to the cafeteria myself. When we get there we sit down at a long table with several Spanish-speaking families with kids of various abilities. Every now and then Evan's alarm beeps and one little girl at our table gets very excited. I check the vent and say,

'Everything's okay' and everyone smiles the tired, weary smiles that parents wear every day around here.

After I finish my pumpkin pie I wheel Evan around to the huge fish tank in the lobby and sit and tell him what each fish looks like. Then I promise him a fish tank when we get back to Scotland (I had no idea how calming it is to watch fish swim).

This evening Evan treats me to a rare run of breathing on his own. He lasts about twenty minutes. I sit and watch every breath.

3 December 2012

Angela R really likes Evan's music set-up and I said I would leave it for her to give to another child. I recently sent out some emails asking friends if they had any old iPods and speakers they would like to donate. Angela R mentioned they are always very low on socks in the playroom, so I added a request for socks (which I highlighted and underlined for emphasis).

Today we have two carts loaded up with seventeen iPods and seventeen speakers (many are new) and 475 pairs of socks, neatly divided by age and size. There are a load of books and toys too, as well as a decent amount of good old-fashioned dollar bills. Angela R is delighted.

5 December 2012

EVAN'S DISCHARGE DATE!

Jackie helped me take our personal belongings back to Manhattan a few days ago, and I have mostly said my goodbyes at the Cabin, the Deli and the garages, so when I wake up this morning all I really have to do is say goodbye to the staff. The therapists all come by to see Evan one last time and a couple of them are more than a little teary.

Then in comes SW2. I've felt our relationship to be a little frayed around the edges recently – probably because I didn't think she was doing enough to speed up our discharge and I let her know it. She comes into our room with a bunch of papers and a lot of information, none of which I can really take in. Then she says, 'Everyone is really sorry about this, but by New York law we have to make every parent watch a video about Shaken Baby Syndrome before their child can be discharged.'

I know she is right. When I was in hospital having Evan I had to watch it. I remember it well: the innocent smiling faces of little babies, and the stories that followed, of shaking and brain damage, and cerebral palsy and sometimes death. I don't need to be reminded of any of this. The nurse brings in the DVD player and sets it up.

'I'm really sorry about this,' she keeps saying. Then she leaves me alone.

I turn the volume down and lower the screen until it is almost closed. Watching it would be one agony too many.

Part Four

Two Weeks in the Apartment

After almost ten months in various hospitals, Evan is finally discharged. He comes back to Manhattan, not to our old apartment, but to this larger, darker place, two floors higher up in the same building, and with a living room as my bedroom and Evan's room a scary jumble of machines, medical supplies, half-packed bags and a Christmas tree I have put together in exuberance at his return.

His machines are basically the same as the ones he had at the hospital. The only difference is that because we don't have an endless supply of oxygen in tanks at home we have been given an oxygen compressor. It's the size and shape of a suitcase on wheels and generates a supply of oxygen via a tube attached to the vent, which is then attached (as it always is) to Evan.

I Believe in Evan

The ambulance gurney can only get as far as our front doorway, and so Evan is carried, in the sitting position, across the threshold in the arms of one of the paramedics that have driven us home. His head is sunken down to his chest, his arms still stuck rigidly to his side with the spasticity he hasn't lost since the early days.

As much as I feel tears of sadness in my eyes I still try to acknowledge the magnitude of the moment. Recognition is certainly due, after all the months we have been through, all the worry that we would never come home together again, that here at last is a little victory for Team Schwarz.

There is little time for sentiment, though. Two nurses and two representatives from the nursing agency are already here, and set to, organising the equipment, reviewing rotas, explaining documents to me and getting me to sign them.

There's a maintenance guy at our apartment building, Mike, who always asks me how Evan is. When I told him a few months ago that he was doing better his eyes filled with tears. 'Oh, thank God,' he said, 'thank God!' When I started to feel anxious about what people's reactions to Evan would be when I got him home, Mike was one of my main concerns. Once Evan is in the apartment and the nurses are settling him in, I go out to get coffee. I pass Mike in the hallway.

'Hey, you're back! Is the baby home?' he asks.

'Yes, he is – the door's open – go in and say hi.'

He says he will. This is a really good move. I don't have to watch Mike's reaction as he sees Evan for the first time. For all I know, it is easier on Mike too. Half an hour later I see him in the hallway again.

Two Weeks in the Apartment

'Oh my God, he's even more beautiful!' he says. 'He's gonna get there, he is. Tell me what you need fixed in your apartment, anything at all, I'll fix it right away.'

I could have kissed him.

By contrast, another maintenance guy spends a lot of time looking away when around Evan. Once, in our apartment, I see him shake his head. A lot. He isn't being mean – he seems to be just showing his angst. I really don't like it at all.

Eventually the first day draws to a close and the nurses and maintenance guys leave and Evan and I are allowed a few hours on our own until the night shift arrives. It is bliss. We lie on the couch together, me cupping his little body in my arms, feeling his warmth, holding him, without the threat of a nurse or doctor walking in, talking to him, without feeling self-conscious at being overheard. We savour even the novelty of the door between us and the outside world being closed.

When the night nurse knocks on the front door a few hours later, Evan and I are still in the same position on the couch. I pick him up and place him in his crib, and then go to answer the door. Almost immediately Evan starts desatting. I run back in and try to work out what is happening. The nurse follows me. I ambu-bag Evan a few times and his sats come back up. Then I put him back on the vent and they fall again. I suction and suction in between more bagging, but his sats keep falling. I know I am going to have to do an emergency trach change. The nurse is standing closer to the spare trach tubes than I am, so I have to tell her where to look, what to grab to give me. She hasn't been in the apartment more than three minutes at this stage so it's a big ask. Eventually I do an emergency trach change. Still no improvement. I look away in despair. And then I see it: the tubing between the oxygen compressor and the vent has become detached. I must have kicked it out when I put Evan back in the crib. I re-attach it and his sats shoot back up to a hundred.

I turn to the nurse and apologise for the drama, and for having barked orders at her. She gives a kind of grunt and takes her coat off. I'm almost certain I hear her curse under her breath.

In the night shifts that follow this particular nurse's attitude doesn't improve, and I feel uneasy about going to sleep. The last straw is when I catch her fast asleep on the couch.

That was the end of that.

Her night shift was taken over by a tall young male nurse, Johnny. He started with us on the day shift. As much as falling asleep on the job can't be tolerated, I am aware that beggars can't be choosers, and even if I personally have reservations about any particular nurse, I have to work through it, so long as they are safe with and good for Evan. Johnny certainly tests this hypothesis.

He tells me he grew up in The Bronx. His accent is all-American that first day. The second day, however, having apparently taken a liking for my Scottish accent, he turns up sporting a Londonesque accent – 'Brilliant, yeah?' he offers at the slightest of opportunities. It's not the first time that I've heard an American go British on me when they hear my accent, so I opt to ignore it. I grit my teeth and get on with the packing. Then, a few days in, he decides that wearing slippers in the apartment (as all the nurses do) isn't enough, so he takes off his shoes and socks and walks around barefoot. Yuck! I keep my shoes on at all possible times after this. Then he starts singing in a high-pitched voice. This stretches me close to the limits. Then he starts putting his size twelve trainers under my bed, right below where my head goes. This pretty much throws me over the edge. It is at this point, thankfully, that he gets switched to nights and I don't have to listen to him, or see him much at all. He is perfectly competent with Evan, and that is really all that matters.

The other nurses are trouble-free, nice to talk to, and very good with Evan. One in particular stands out, not least because, on a doctor's visit, Evan started desatting in the ambulance and she handled the whole thing with total professionalism and calm. I ask her if she is willing to make the journey to Scotland with us and she is.

Of course, the two-week transition period to the portable vent (which Dr M had insisted on before we can take Evan on a plane) is not without further drama.

On day four of being home, the night nurse wakes me to tell me she is worried Evan has an infection. We call an ambulance. By the time it comes, Johnny, who is still on day shifts, arrives to take over, and comes with us to the emergency room.

We haven't been in this particular hospital before. We are wheeled into a curtained area, where Evan is hooked up to the hospital monitor and given regular oxygen. A nice young male doctor examines him and, very reassuringly, tells me that he will 'do everything in my power to ensure Evan does not get admitted to hospital'. He explains at length that hospitals have lots of germs running up and down the bed frames, on doors, in chairs, wherever you can think of, and that he doesn't want to subject Evan to that risk. I don't bother explaining that Evan, as he should know, has just done a ten-month stint in one and that if anyone has built a good immune system it is him. Once the young male doctor leaves the room, Johnny, apropos of absolutely nothing, says, 'Doctors can be very arrogant.' I really don't need a second opinion so I give Johnny the rest of the day off.

After about five hours of hardly anything at all happening, the young male doctor comes back in to our curtained area with a female doctor, who tells us Evan is indeed being admitted to hospital, and an ambulance will be taking us back to Columbia ICU in the next half hour.

Thanks a bunch, Dr Wetbehindtheears.

By this time I know that Evan is actually doing just fine again, but I most definitely am not going to argue against hospitalisation. I know enough by now to let the doctors make their own mistakes, so long as Evan is not being neglected.

In the meantime, though, we are about an hour late for Evan's blood pressure medication. I made this known about three hours earlier. I didn't think we would be there for more than an hour or two and haven't brought his evening meds with us. I tell the female doctor that this is becoming an issue and she assures me she will get meds from the pharmacy. Another hour passes.

There are probably only six or eight curtained bays like ours in this section, but there clearly isn't enough staff to cover all of them. In the hallway between the bays many parents are walking up and down, sick of waiting, although they haven't been waiting nearly as long as us.

Eventually our ambulance arrives and two burly New Yorkers in paramedic uniforms come and started strapping Evan onto their cart, bantering away with me, jovially nagging at each other. I tell them they are like an old married couple. 'He's the wife,' they both say in unison, pointing at the other.

They set to, getting all the paperwork completed and Evan's equipment checked against their own. All seems okay until they take his blood pressure. 'That ain't that baby's,' says one to the other. I take a look. The systolic is up at 200, and the diastolic is at 140.

'That's his,' I say, with growing concern. I tell them how long we have been waiting for the meds.

'Let's just take him to Columbia and they can sort him out there,' says one.

'Nah,' says the other. 'If he keeps rising like this, he ain't gonna make it to Columbia.'

There is only one thing for it. I stand in the hallway outside our bay and start shouting, 'His blood pressure is up at 200! How high does it have to get before he gets his medicine?'

I don't let up until it has its effect. Immediately the female doctor appears and a couple of paramedics emerge from another bay (leaving behind their newspapers, but no patient, despite the impression the closed curtain had given). There is much hustle and bustling all of a sudden, albeit almost entirely carried out with an ill will. But I get what I want. Evan's medication had apparently been prepared already and has been sitting in a loaded syringe on a nearby trolley for an hour and a half, with no one taking any further responsibility for it.

The nurse that rushes in with it stops to give me a dirty look and then begins to inject it into Evan's gastro-tube.

'Don't give me that look,' I warn her. 'This is my son and you'd better look after him.'

'Shouting isn't going to help any,' she says, in a softened tone.

'Shouting is the only thing that has helped,' I snarl back.

I have no doubt they are all very glad to see us leave. Me too.

I dread going back to Columbia ICU. The worst month of our lives was spent there. I mostly fear someone saying, 'See, he isn't any better. We told you that you should have withdrawn care.'

We are taken back to the ninth floor. It doesn't feel so bad to be back after all. There is a familiarity about the place. As a matter of fact, it actually feels comforting to be here.

Dr Patrick, the handsome red-haired doctor who had used the crash cart to stabilise Evan on that second night, is on duty. He looks genuinely pleased to see us. I recognise most of the nurses. The nurse assigned to Evan tells me to call up a friend, and go out for dinner and a few drinks.

'I want my own quiet time with Mr Evan,' she smiles.

I call Deborah and we meet in the Irish bar on the corner. After an hour or so I come back to Evan, make up my little bed beside his, and go to sleep.

I suppose our return to the ICU is a good measure of how far we have come these past ten months. The noises of the machines and alarms aren't scary at all any more. I know pretty much everything that is going on with Evan and I don't carry the horrendous fear of the new and unknown like I did before. As a matter of fact, now I kind of like showing off my confidence in Evan.

It's also nice to see the staff again. Most of the nurses worked here back in February and they all want to see Evan's wavy hair and to ooh and aah about how much he has grown. Music therapy Kate stops by and we have a huge hug before she plays Evan a few songs on her guitar.

I bump into Dr Brown.

'I wanted to reach out, to keep in touch,' she tells me, 'but I felt with the criminal case against the babysitter, it wouldn't really be appropriate.' There is some sadness in her voice.

'I absolutely understood that,' I tell her, adding, 'I'm in a much better place now.'

'Yes, I can see that,' she says, the twinkle returning to her eye.

I even see the medium devil doctor – the neurologist with the satchel. He is examining the patient next to Evan. His colleague is haranguing him for some misstep he has apparently taken recently. He is looking tired and his skin has lost the healthy sheen it had back in February.

The neighbourhood has changed a little. A couple of restaurants have shut down; none have replaced them yet. On the street is an entertainer of sorts, who I remember but hadn't the chance to enjoy during our last visit. He is a forty-something African-American wearing tight pants, a shiny sequined silver top, sunglasses and large headphones, with a microphone in his hand. The microphone is attached to nothing, but he twirls and dances around the pavement, talking into it as though he is a Diva doing a soundcheck. ('I need more lights on me, more lights on me.') Brilliant! I've never seen this guy asking for money so I presume he does it purely for pleasure.

After two nights we are once again set free and Evan and I return to our temporary space on 71st Street. The routine with the nurses continues and things are calm enough for me to get Evan and me ready for the move back to Scotland.

As well as packing our clothes, I have to organise Evan's equipment. I know we won't be allowed to carry oxygen on board the plane, and so I have to arrange for a special portable oxygen compressor that runs on batteries and will fit beneath the seat in front.

I also have to organise the apartment a little. The movers I have hired are going to come in and pack everything up once we leave, but I still have to make sure everything is in order for them. The busy-ness of the task of leaving helps to alleviate some of the nerves already gathering about the flight home with Evan.

Somewhere in the midst of all this I hear from the anti-ACS attorneys. It turns out it won't be worthwhile suing ACS after all. The first reason is that as soon as ACS got the Grimm Report they dismissed the case against me. Apparently there is some legal precedent that says before there is medical evidence to the contrary they can bring charges against anyone remotely connected to the child. The second reason is that I signed the consent form referring Evan to a long-term facility. I explained to them my reasons for this, that I felt I had no choice, but it doesn't matter. I signed it, which implies I agreed with the move (even though I didn't).

I feel relieved. I don't want to expend the energy it would take to sue ACS. It would cause more bad feeling and more anxiety, lawsuits always do. And I need all my energy for Evan.

Four days before we are due to fly home, once again Evan ends up back in hospital. The problem is basically the same as the week before: he is desatting and the nurse and I can't work out why. She calls an ambulance, but the crew we are sent have no ventilator experience. We end up having to transport Evan detached from the vent, ambuing him all the way.

Getting out of the apartment building during the morning rush is a task in itself. We have to politely ask an entire elevator full of people to vacate on our floor so we can take it downstairs without delay. They are very willing to oblige, but the looks on their faces when they see this tiny boy lying motionless on a stretcher, having air bagged into him, doesn't do much to reduce my own stress. Still, we get him to the ER. This time we go to Cornell, which is on the east side of the city, and has its own paediatric ICU, which means we won't have to be transported anywhere else if Evan has to be admitted.

Once we are in the ER, Evan is placed in yet another cubicle and attached to yet another set of hospital machines.

When the doctor arrives the nurse tries to 'present' Evan's case to him but is getting confused so I step in.

'He is vent-dependent 24/7, oxygen dependent to twenty-five per cent, tachycardic, hypertensive, g-tube fed. Today he had sudden drops in his saturation levels. Ambuing restored but back on the vent he desatted several more times and an ambulance was called and he was brought here.'

The doctor thanks me and asks, 'Are you a medical professional?'

'No, but I've lived in a couple of hospitals,' I reply.

Later, the doctor takes me into the hallway and asks me what happened to Evan originally. I try to hold back the tears but I just can't. How I hate having to explain the diagnosis every single time we meet a new doctor.

When we get back into the cubicle and I see Evan I start screaming at the nurses.

'He's not on the vent! He needs to be ventilated 24/7!'

'Well, he's breathing fine on his own,' one of them replies, looking slightly puzzled.

And so he is, little Evan the wonder boy is breathing on his own with nothing but a tiny little oxygen mask held to his trach opening. He is satting beautifully – I can't believe it.

After about twenty minutes or so his breaths get too weak and he has to go back on the vent. Then things start to go awry: he starts desatting no matter how much oxygen is being pumped into him. Eventually, the decision is made to transport him upstairs to the ICU, ambuing him all the way in case the problem lies with the ventilator.

It's a very nervy elevator trip to the sixth floor.

Evan is brought into a room with six doctors, a respiratory therapist and two nurses. One doctor, a young Nigerian woman, takes charge. She works out that Evan's right lung has collapsed.

Two Weeks in the Apartment

She has a complex discussion with the respiration therapist, does some calculations and then, very swiftly, adjusts a setting on Evan's vent (called the 'peep') up to its maximum, in six short spurts. The effect is that Evan's lung becomes re-inflated in a slow and steady manner. Within ten minutes he is back to normal. I fall in love with the doctor.

They decide to keep Evan in overnight to make sure he really has recovered. I sleep by his bed again, this time with a view of the East River and the FDR Drive, where a stream of cars passes under our window all night long.

We are discharged the next day around noon (although the ambulance doesn't arrive to take us home until 10pm).

I spend the remaining few days packing, saying goodbye to people and wondering, briefly, if leaving New York is the right thing to do.

I make two lists:

1. Reasons to Stay in New York or at Least to Come Back to New York One Day:

   A. I have wonderful friends here and these past ten months have deepened our friendships.
   B. I love the clear air and cloudless skies over the Upper West Side in the winter evenings.
   C. I can't dig deep enough to find a third reason right now.

2. Reasons to Leave New York and Not to Think About Coming Back Until I am Ready, Which is Not Now:

I Believe in Evan

A. Every time I cross the street between the subway and my apartment I remember running to the first ambulance on 18 January 2012. I walk to the deli past the photo shop and I remember putting my hand in my pocket, pulling out my phone and reading the text that would tear through our happiness on 17 February 2012. I walk back to the apartment and I remember the terrifying run I made that day, not knowing what I would find in the apartment.

B. Even though I changed apartments, whenever I go through the lobby I remember running in and running out. I remember Norma's words, 'They can't get a pulse' and the lady on the phone, 'Your son is very, very sick'. I remember frantically trying to get a cab.

C. It's just too painful to stay in Manhattan for now. I have too many unhappy memories from the last ten months (which right now have overtaken some wonderful memories of the last ten years).

D. New York will always be here.

It's not about doing the right thing – going back to Scotland is really the only thing I can do right now. Whatever happens, my future is with Evan. I don't know what that entails, but I'm grateful for the opportunity. Whatever happens, I will leave this world, many years from now, knowing that I did everything I possibly could to give my son the best life he could have.

Part Five

Back in Glasgow

Two weeks after we make it out of Blythedale we are ready to leave for Scotland. The luggage begins to pile up. We have two suitcases of clothes, a portable oxygen compressor, a bag with batteries, a bag with blood pressure machine and nebuliser (to steam liquid medicine through the ventilator), a pulse-ox machine, a portable suction machine, a food pump, food, ventilator, pushchair, car seat. The nurse busies herself checking and rechecking everything. I do a lot of nervous pacing.

My cousin Madeleine comes to say goodbye. During these past few months I have spent a lot of time with her. I will miss her as much as I will miss anyone or anything in New York. Her husband Dave arrives to help us out to the ambulance and he and the nurse travel together in a car with all the luggage, while Evan and I travel in the ambulance, ahead of them.

En route, Pamela Turner calls. She wants to know if she can come and see Evan. ACS has absolutely no authority over either of us any more, but her nameless, faceless supervisor apparently wants her to visit us. I tell her we are on our way to the airport. 'Which one?' she asks. Is she really going to come and see us at the airport? I am not prepared to take the risk of being upset by her any more. 'JFK,' I tell her, just as the ambulance takes the exit towards Newark airport.

Newark Airport Security is notoriously busy and stressful at the best of times, but being so close to Christmas I expected it to be worse than usual. When we get to the kerbside of the departures terminal, the ambulance and car are both emptied of Evan's things and it all lies on the pavement with Evan in his pushchair in the middle of it. There is organised chaos all around us. Dave finds an airport employee who comes along with a large cart and we all set about putting everything on it. We get into the terminal and up to the check-in desk and the employee bids us farewell but waits for a tip, which he gets.

At the check-in desk I ask for assistance getting through security. A short, stocky lady in an airport uniform arrives with a two-way radio and spends at least twenty minutes trying to page someone to come and help us.

'No one likes doing the disabled runs,' she says with too much candour.

I am getting sick and tired of waiting so I tell her that Evan's batteries are about to run out. That lights a fire under her and she takes us through herself. (I am aware that I have told two white lies within a short space of time and wonder what Mr Polygraph would make of that.)

We form a caravan of equipment and people for our trek through Newark Airport Security. The airport employee leads, pushing our oversized trolley of luggage, followed by Evan in his oversized pushchair with vent attached, followed by me pushing him and then the nurse following behind us with the oxygen compressor, attached by a long connector to Evan's ventilator, and with several bags. We bypass the snaking lines of bored travellers all waiting with their passports at the ready, all with nothing to do but stare at us. It isn't pleasant, but it is over quickly as we are swarmed by eight blue-shirted airport security employees, who politely bring us past the X-ray machines and one by one go over each and every item of luggage or equipment we have. All we have to do is sit and wait for them to be done. It is quick and it holds as little stress as is possible in the circumstances. Getting on to the plane isn't rough either. We are allowed to board well ahead of everyone else and given time to get ourselves settled, with all the equipment in place before the able-bodied masses join us.

The nurse and I are ecstatic to see that the plane has electrical sockets for every seat. We had been told it was a possibility but there was no guarantee. We find a socket for every plug of every machine we have and congratulate ourselves that we won't have to worry about using up the remaining battery power.

About ten minutes after take-off we realise one machine is working off battery anyway. Then another. And another. It turns out that the plane's sockets aren't designed for the massive rush of voltage they experience when we plug all of Evan's machines in at the same time. We have not only blown the sockets that we are using, but, because they are all connected in circuit lines running up and down the cabin, we have blown every single socket on our side of the plane: we are back to batteries. We let the cabin crew know that we are slightly concerned that we will run out of power, but are reassured that, if we do, Evan can go and sit in the cockpit with the pilot who, apparently, has an impervious electrical socket that never fails. The steward takes the extra step of having a word with the pilot, who contacts Air Traffic Control and makes sure our plane won't be delayed in any way at all, as Evan is on board and fast using up batteries. We don't run out of battery power, but a picture of Evan in the cockpit would have been priceless.

When I am not monitoring the batteries I am staring at Evan's monitors. His oxygen levels stay well above ninety per cent the entire way. In fact he looks remarkably comfortable throughout the flight. Perhaps he knows we are going home, or maybe it's just the hum of the plane's engines.

When the plane lands we still have plenty of battery power, so we wait until every passenger is off the plane before getting our massive haul together. The stewards all hang around helping, lifting bags, guiding wires. I see one surreptitiously wipe a tear away. I wish she'd do it openly – I could tell her it was all going to be just fine.

Once off the plane, a couple of ground-crew guys help us from the gate through Customs and out into the fresh Glasgow air. It's a long walk, and they push two overloaded carts for us all the way from the plane, through Customs, to baggage and out to the taxi. I hand them a twenty. 'No, hen, don't be daft!' they say. I make them take it anyway.

We take a taxi for the final part of the journey. When we arrive at Yorkhill hospital the driver gets out and goes to find a couple of porters to help us. Not long after, we are in a ward with other ventilated babies, and a lot of fuss around us.

Evan's new bed is by the window on the fifth floor. He has a view of the River Clyde. As soon as I lay him down, he looks more relaxed than I have ever seen him. Both arms feel much less constricted than their tone usually allows. It is as if he is delighted to have made it here.

As he sleeps comfortably in his new surroundings, I am taken through the intake procedure with the doctors and nurses. I know Evan's medical notes have already been forwarded from Blythedale to Yorkhill, but I still have to explain everything all over again. Once I have done all that, a very gentle nurse comes to see me with a new-looking binder that is to be Evan's medical file for the ward.

'What would you like me to write down as the diagnosis?' she asks, in a lilting accent.

'It's Shaken Baby Syndrome,' I say once again, now almost numbed to the pain of saying it out loud.

'Yes, but we could just put traumatic brain injury if you would prefer – would that be easier for you?'

I could have kissed her. In all this time it hasn't occurred to me or to anyone else that it might be kinder to give Evan's condition a more sterile description.

Eventually, the paperwork is complete, Evan is well settled and in good hands, and I can go home to sleep off a little jet lag.

I have an emotional meeting with Mum. We hug in her hallway for an age. She is delighted to finally have company, after living alone in the now oversized family home (it used to hold Mum, Dad and five kids) for the last year and a half, since Dad died. I am delighted to be back in the comfort and warmth of it all: it feels very safe.

There's a holly tree in Mum's front garden. Once the third of three trees (the large and the small silver birches being the other two), it is now the only one remaining. It stands just at the wall between her garden and the neighbours'. Its leaves are variegated with a blond tip. I still remember my feeling of pride at the age of seven when our holly was chosen to adorn the Christmas wreath at school because it was the most unusual. The poor holly tree doesn't look too good right now. Its top two-thirds have been hacked off. Not as hacked off as I am. Apparently, while Evan and I were in Blythedale, the neighbour was concerned that the tree's roots were affecting his garage floor. Mum hadn't wanted it to become an issue so without any coaxing from the neighbour, and having taken absolutely no advice from any professional, she just allowed someone with a chainsaw to have a go at it. Seeing this once stunning tree reduced to half its size, with just a canopy of branches, mostly bald and spiderish, makes me feel immeasurably sad. I actually can't get it out of my mind. I really don't know why I have developed such an emotional attachment to these trees, especially when I have so much else going on.

Back in Glasgow

Evan's ward has eight single rooms and three larger shared rooms. His bed is in a six-bed bay and four of the other five babies in the bay have tracheostomies. Three are ventilator dependent too, just like Evan. Each of these five children has at least one family member sitting with them for most of the day. There is always at least one nurse in the room at all times, but there are usually two or three. The nursing station is just a few feet away, and there is always some kind of doctor around, as well as a handful of support staff. The atmosphere is cheery and friendly.

The walls are painted with colourful murals, but the building itself is a little rundown. The entire children's hospital is preparing for a move to the south side of the city in two years' time. From Evan's window you can actually see the new building being built across the river. For now, though, our surroundings are not state of the art, as Blythedale's were. That's no deal breaker in our situation. Now that we are finally 'home' and the stress of the journey is behind us, I am starting to feel strong gratitude that we made it here.

A few things, however, are obvious improvements on life at Blythedale. The 'code blue' rapid response procedure that terrorised us there isn't used here. I watched a nurse attend a little girl at her hospital bed today. The nurse needed assistance, so she tugged on a red lever above the girl's bed. I didn't hear any alarm sound, but within seconds three nurses had arrived, walking quickly, not running, and not panicking. Whatever the problem had been was taken care of, and everyone went back to what they were doing. The room didn't fill with all the staff in the building, there was no excess anxiety, and there was no lengthy comedown from the experience. Blythedale could learn a thing or two here.

For me the biggest difference is probably the fact that there isn't the facility to sleep next to Evan's bed. Parents who come from farther away can take a room in the guesthouse down the street from the hospital, but it makes more sense for me to stay with my mum, who lives just a few miles away. Selfishly, I think that's great. If I could stay by Evan's side twenty-four hours a day I would, but I can't, and the thought of getting a full night's sleep in a real bed, large and soft, in a quiet house and waking up refreshed and ready to make the short journey to see him every day is exceptionally appealing.

24 December 2012

CHRISTMAS EVE

Evan looks awful. His vent settings were changed today. Apparently the volumes he was on are 'shocking' by British standards, so the consultant, Dr Davies, reset them to more acceptable levels. Unfortunately this hospital has yet to learn that Evan doesn't follow anyone's rules but his own. The new settings leave him grey and gasping. Thankfully I arrive not long after the change has been made, but there is a stressful half hour or so until the consultant finds his way back and changes the settings back again (which only he can do). Naturally, I give him a good piece of my mind. ('Who the hell do you think you are?' etc.) Dr Davies is extremely apologetic. Maybe he thinks we've got off to a bad start. Actually, so long as Evan is okay, I think it's quite a good start from my point of view. It's no bad thing for them to know that I will make an uncomfortable scene if I think for one second that Evan's needs aren't being properly met.

25 December 2012

CHRISTMAS DAY

I wake up at 5am, wishing Evan was with me. I have to wait for Mum to wake up, so I can take her to see him at the hospital. As soon as she does, I make her a hasty breakfast of scrambled eggs and smoked salmon and then we set off. I can't get there fast enough – I just want to be with my boy on Christmas Day.

Mum and Evan have a lovely cuddle. She holds him, touching his face, stroking his hair. He purrs. As I watch them, I remember the feeling I had, not so very long ago, that they would never see each other again.

Dr Davies comes by to wish us a Merry Christmas. He doesn't seem to harbour any ill feeling about yesterday and I am impressed.

Once he leaves, Mum asks, 'Who was the doctor you were shouting at yesterday?'

'That's him.'

'What, that lovely young man? But he's so nice!'

One of the nurses overhears Mum. She had been on duty yesterday and knows all about it.

'Phil? He is nice, actually,' she says, almost apologetically to me. 'He never loses his temper and he's really nice to the nurses and parents.'

In the spirit of Christmas I decide to let bygones be bygones. I also feel a bit mean for having been so hard on him. Evan is still a bit grey after yesterday, though, so I only need to look at him to remind myself that it's my job to fight for his best interests, not to make anyone else feel okay.

Another change to Blythedale practice is that everyone here calls the doctors by their first names. But I'm not falling for that one. I'm not going to get all pally-wally with 'Phil' and then one day be asked to sit down with him, like two old friends, while he tells me terrible things about Evan I don't want to hear. I'm fine with keeping salutations and awkward distances, thank you very much.

26 December 2012

The lighting in the ward is very different than at Blythedale. The walls and curtains are blue and the ceiling is grey, but the outside light is very dull right now too as the weather is stormy and dark, even in daylight. As a result I can't really tell if Evan looks so grey because of the vent change two days ago, or if it's just the reflection of the colours around him. As well as this, his eyes have become red and sore looking due to a mixture of the change in environment and the different eye ointment they use here. The end result is that he looks like something out of *The Exorcist*.

2 January 2013

As I get ready to leave home for the hospital this morning I get a call from the ward.

'Is everything okay?' I ask before the nurse finishes speaking.

'No,' she says, 'Evan isn't well. We think he has sepsis.'

I run out of the house and drive as fast as I can to the hospital. It's still a holiday here so the roads are quiet. On the way I try researching 'sepsis' on my phone. I don't have time to stop and read the results and the only words I can make out as I drive along are 'life threatening' and 'death'.

I run into the ward to find the curtains pulled around Evan's bed. The nurse is looking very anxious. I pull the curtains back and see Evan, bright red and writhing, with his ventilator alarming 'high pressure' at a furious rate.

I feel instantly relieved.

'That's what he does when he's teething,' I tell them. 'We usually give him a painkiller and he settles down in an hour.'

A doctor appears and we talk.

'You might be right, and I hope you are,' he tells me when I tell him about the teething, 'but we need to do a thorough investigation into this.'

He sends Evan's blood off for various tests and tells the nurses to carry out more frequent sets of observation on him. I sit and hold Evan as he writhes some more. Sure enough, after an hour or so he settles down. It dawns on me that giving him a painkiller and hoping that this will solve the problem – as we had always believed at Blythedale – might not actually be the answer. Just because the Blythedale doctors didn't offer any kind of solution doesn't mean there isn't a solution available.

7 January 2013

The neurologist comes to see me on the ward today. She leads with, 'You don't need me to tell you Evan has had a devastating injury.'

No, and I really don't need her to remind me of it either. She talks about the writhing and high-pressuring we had seen a few days before. The tests have shown Evan does not have sepsis, but the neurologist is still worried about the symptoms. She has decided to start him on a drug called chlorpromazine. She explains that it is a neurologically based medication, but there's no guarantee as to whether it will regulate the parts of the brain that need regulating.

'Sometimes it's more art than science,' she says.

I don't enjoy the conversation but I do feel good about having sat and listened to it head-on. I also feel relieved that there is actually something that might help Evan.

Later, when Evan is settled and lying in my arms again, he poops with such gusto that I drop my book.

Back in Glasgow

3 January 2013

I have an appointment at the Job Centre today to see about collecting unemployment benefits. I used to be a New York lawyer. I had a thriving practice, and an office so high up in a downtown Manhattan building that I could see both rivers. I had an Upper West Side apartment, a brownstone in Brooklyn and a pension plan. I had a healthy baby boy. And we had two doctors and a babysitter.

A nice lady tells me to take a seat at her desk and works her way through a series of computerised questionnaires.

No, I'm not working.

Yes, I have one child.

No, I don't own or rent.

I live with my mother in her house.

My child doesn't live with me right now.

My sorry life story falls on fiscally deaf ears. I am told I have to wait until I've been a UK resident for a full six months before I qualify for government assistance. I slope off back under the rock that has engulfed my life.

I leave the Job Centre and walk through Shawlands towards the bus that will take me to Evan. On the way, I stop at a shop in Shawlands arcade to look for a set of headphones for him. Because there are so many people around his bed now, including other patients, we can't play his music on a speaker any more. The only headphones I find that I can afford have an arm with a microphone attached. I buy them and take them to Evan. I put them on him, and attach them to his iPod. Then I hold him while I read a magazine. Every now and then I lower the arm so it looks like he is either in telesales or about to start singing.

The redness of Evan's eyes (from the change in environment) has turned into a bad eye infection. It has been treated with strong medication. The infection is gone now but has left scratches on his cornea. The left one, in particular, is quite noticeable: it's a white horizontal line, against his big blue iris.

When his eyes are open he still can't blink, which means he can't lubricate them naturally. So he has to have eye drops every two hours. A bigger problem, though, is that, when he sleeps, his eyes don't close fully; there is always a bit of blue showing. The left eye is slightly worse than the right one. The air gets in and dries them out some more. This worsens the scratch and could lead to another infection. So, at night-time he gets his eyes taped shut with blue medical tape.

When I leave him this evening I make sure the blue tape is on properly. Then I lower the microphone arm to his mouth again, before propping him up on either side with various soft toys so he is comfortable. The oversized head of a long bright green serpent snake cuddles into him, its big red tongue almost licking his face, protectively. I imagine the nurses laughing when they see him like this.

9 January 2013

I walk in alongside another mother in our ward today and we start a conversation. It has taken me this long to realise that, being number four on the list for home care, our three remaining neighbours are actually numbers one, two and three. I preferred the anonymity of our competition. It's more difficult to wish yourself ahead of another mother and child when you know and like them.

All three babies are around a year old. They were all born at least two months prematurely. Each has a tracheostomy and is vent dependent to varying degrees. Number One is the lone girl. She likes to flirt with everyone and has a chubby little face that is impossible not to smile at. Number Two cries when Number One stops paying him attention. Number Three has a smile that is so big it almost meets itself behind the back of his head. All three are active little things, but because of the way their tracheostomy tubes sit, none of them can make any oral sounds.

In the last few weeks Evan has increased his ability to make phonating sounds. Because his throat and mouth (and face) are still entirely paralysed, he has limited control over when (only with the outward flow of air) and how he makes these noises. His little voice box has to do all the work alone. But that is enough for him to be able to convey in his tone whether he is happy ('uhr, uhr, uhr, uhr') or upset ('ug, ug, ug, ug'). All of this to say my little Evan is the noisy one on the ward.

10 January 2013

Because I can't sleep at the hospital now I have lots of free time. Because I'm happier here than I was in New York, I also have more energy than I had before. I've been out of Glasgow for too long to know how to spend either, and I'm also not quite ready to face the public yet. As a solution, I've started decorating my mum's house. My mum isn't as pleased about this as I would have expected. Every evening I come home and strip another bit of wallpaper off or sand something. It feels great to be active after almost a year of inertia. Tonight I am stripping paint off the wainscoting in the bathroom, decade upon decade of various colours and textures. The smell is a little overpowering, and I end up knee deep in half-burnt paint shavings, but it's a terrific distraction.

I finish around 2am and go downstairs for a cup of tea. As I sit at the kitchen table I suddenly hear Mum rush from her bedroom into the hall, shouting, 'Where are you?' She says she heard me shouting at her to get up, that something was 'urgent'. I tell her everything is fine and it must have been a dream. She laughs it off and goes back to bed. I hope she isn't getting the same nightmares I get. I don't know if I should explain to her how I have come to adjust to having a horrific, stressful dream every single night and maybe she is going to have to do the same. She's back in bed now; she won't sleep, though. Tomorrow she will say to me, 'I didn't sleep a wink all night, and when I woke up I was exhausted.' It's a running joke.

12 January 2013

My birthday. I spend most of today crying. 'Happy' occasions have that effect on me these days. Friends come over this evening. I have too much to drink. I run off to the park in the dark and lie under a tree, hoping to fall asleep and just be taken by God. Then it starts raining and I come back home.

15 January 2013

I feel awful. I went into an Indian restaurant tonight and ordered takeaway food. As I waited for my order, my eye caught a lady sitting having dinner with a friend. Her face was incredibly disfigured. I couldn't work out if it was covered in burns or she had been the victim of a knife attack. Suddenly she looked me right in the eye. I had been staring at her. I couldn't believe I had just done exactly the same rotten thing that annoys me so much when people do it to Evan.

I suppose the moral of this is that people stare. It's not very nice, but it's what we do.

20 January 2013

I'm still getting used to being back in Scotland. There are the obvious differences (driving on the other side of the road, different meanings for certain words) but every now and then, like today when I was called 'Madam' in the supermarket, I get taken aback.

My accent, of course, doesn't stand out here at all. I used to love that in the USA. (Where you from? Scaatlaand?) It was definitely a plus at times. But I had to adjust it ever so slightly when I first became a lawyer just so I could be clearly understood (many will say I never achieved that). When this crisis hit, though, I couldn't keep up the effort and reverted to talking too fast, not rounding the corners of certain words, narrowing my mouth to form words as opposed to widening it (as ten 'accent reduction' lessons in a tiny office next to Grand Central Station had taught me to do), using Scottish colloquialisms that fit my mood better than the Americanisms I had adopted, and forcing people to accommodate me, instead of the other way around.

Given all that, what is now different for me about being in Scotland is that people understand me as soon as I talk. I don't have to wait for the cocked head, momentary-silence-before-response that I had become used to in all those hospitals. It's as if a time-delay issue has finally been resolved: familiarity is wonderful.

My name is a source of confusion here, however. My first and last names have conflicting S's. In New York, Schwarz is a fairly common name, so people usually get at least that part right, even if they fluff on Elise. In Scotland, Schwarz is not common at all. As a result, when I tell Scottish people my name is Elise Schwarz they often give variations, most of which end up sounding like 'Elish Watts'. I don't mind – it might be nice to be someone else for a while.

25 January 2013

I haven't heard from Sergeant Accomando since November. I lost his contact details so I had to do an online search to find him. I found a phone number and some kind of report that said he makes $90,000 a year and gets a bonus of $25,000. I guess he had already qualified for his bonus by the time he and I first spoke. If not then, based on my experience alone, 2012 should have been a lean year for him. I left him a message but I'm still waiting for him to reply.

It annoys me that I have to make the effort. I forgive Norma, because Evan needs me to. I need me to, for that matter. I can't keep moving forward if I am weighed down by negativity for her. But I need the NYPD to do what they are supposed to do, and investigate what happened: to question Norma. To find some answers. I know none of it will help Evan, and in fact it might upset me to hear the truth, but I have an image of me in ten years' time, suddenly engulfed in anger because I have realised that not enough was done for Evan. One of my many fears is that the investigation into how this happened will just fade away.

27 January 2013

Evan hasn't had one of his awful writhing fevered episodes since he started taking the new medication. Also, his heart rate has risen — it was sitting at a worryingly low 50 bpm for weeks, and now it's up to a more regular 125 bpm. His eyes open a lot more often too, and there is more light in them than before. It's a gradual awakening, but it seems the medication is working.

I'm overjoyed at the improvement, but I'm also quite annoyed. All those months at Blythedale, all those times I would see the consultant neurologist sitting having lunch with the staff in the canteen, in his perfectly laundered oversized pink shirts, offering nothing to save my little boy from those awful fits, when all the time there was the possibility of a solution. Yes, my own inertia didn't help, but why didn't they just try a little harder? It makes me mad.

7 February 2013

I had forgotten how hard it is to deal with professional medical opinions. For a while now, I've been the fount of knowledge regarding Evan's health – every doctor that we have met in emergency rooms and at Yorkhill has had to listen to me tell them what's going on with Evan. It's been a lot easier on me. But a few days ago the neurologist at Yorkhill told me she wanted to do a new EEG and MRI so she could establish what is going on neurologically with Evan. I knew it was a bad idea – no doctor has ever looked inside Evan's head and liked what they've seen.

They did both tests two days ago. I thought the EEG might have gone okay because as Evan lay there with wires leading from a computer monitor attached to his head with medical stickers, he did all the things he can do – gave a little squirm, made a tiny noise. As for the MRI – well, I knew that had gone badly because the doctor who performed it had been very chatty and cheery with me before Evan was rolled into the canon. When I came back an hour later, he couldn't look at me. Instead he just kept talking to me through Evan ('We did fine, didn't we, Evan? There was no issue'). I haven't played much poker, but if I had, I would want to play him. Everything about him said this was a bad hand.

Today, the neurologist shows up at Evan's bedside.

'Can we have a meeting about Evan's results?' she asks me.

Back in Glasgow

We go into the family room. I brace myself. A nurse sits beside me, taking notes. The neurologist rubs her forehead. Then she begins talking.

'The EEG isn't flat; there's at least that. But the MRI – in twenty-five years of experience, it's as bad as I've ever seen.'

She explains that she doesn't believe Evan's breathing will ever come back ('The brain stem is too badly damaged') and ends with, 'What do you want to do?'

What I want to do is to punch her in the face. Instead I ask, 'Are you asking me about withdrawing care?'

She looks a bit surprised. 'Well, no, I think we've come too far for that.'

The realisation that this issue is off the table in this hospital is a turning point (it felt like it constantly lurked in the shadows at Blythedale). I tell her that, as far as her diagnosis and prognosis go, she hasn't told me anything new. This, of course, isn't strictly true, but it is enough to ward off the kind of onslaught I had heard from Dr Evil last year. I add that Evan is my son and that my solitary goal is to do as much for him as I possibly can.

'He's precious to you, I understand that,' she replies.

I leave the room and go back to Evan, but I can't stay on the ward any longer. I pick up my coat and bag and leave. I walk down the five flights of stairs to the ground floor of the hospital, leave by the side door, walk down the hill to my car and only then, safely inside, dissolve into tears.

I wish I could hear that kind of news the way I hear driving directions and conversations that include the calculation of numbers – just jumbled words in a white haze, as my thoughts drift away to something else. Instead, though, the words feel sharper than any I have ever heard.

I am still sobbing when I arrive home. Poor Mum thinks there has been a bad change in Evan's condition. The reality is there hasn't been any change at all.

Later in the evening, with my eyes still puffy from all that crying, I go back to the hospital and sit and hold Evan for an hour or so. He is warm and relaxed and I know he can feel me, even though he is asleep. It makes all the difference to me. Holding Evan always does.

10 February 2013

I've had a rough few days. I have experienced a rare patch of anger. Actually, I have felt as much anger as I have been capable of feeling since this happened: angry at Norma, angry at Yorkhill's neurologist, angry at anything, really. It's started to taper off a bit now. I have calmed down enough to remember that you can't fight anger when it comes. You just have to quietly open the door and ask it to leave.

I suppose I first began to feel better when another parent saw me sitting with Evan on the ward and came over to chat to me. Her daughter is ten and fully ventilated, too. Her condition is terminal. The mum didn't try to sugarcoat her daughter's situation and didn't pretend to do the same with Evan's. She had a refreshingly warm realism about her.

'We are the chosen ones,' she told me, smiling, as she was leaving.

Back in Glasgow

25 February 2013

Remember the time back in October when I didn't feel comfortable going to mass because the cardinal had ordered all priests to read out a homophobic letter on the pulpit? Well, that cardinal has just had to resign because it has emerged that he's had numerous homosexual affairs. Homophobes are the biggest closet cases!

10 March 2013

SCOTTISH MOTHER'S DAY!

We have come a long way from last Mother's Day (literally)! When I came to the ward today I was given a delightful poster with Evan's hands imprinted in red paint. The ward staff had helped him make it. I love being a mum! Later, my lovely friend Emma arrived, holding something behind her back. She told me to shut my eyes and, when I opened them again, Evan had a card and a present in his hand for his mummy! It was so sweet. Emma was a single mother herself for a very long time and has made it a habit to organise Evan with a present for me on suitable occasions.

I Believe in Evan

30 March 2013

EASTER SUNDAY

Evan Louis Schwarz is christened at St Gabriel's RC Church in Merrylee, Glasgow today. Friends and family come from far and wide – from Ireland, England, New York, Spain and Germany. Violet and Neil B are lovely godparents. My mum cries at the service (she never cries). I swear once in the church when Evan's vent becomes disconnected briefly (the priest gives me instant forgiveness upon request). I am so incredibly proud of my boy. This is the second happiest day of my life (after the day of his birth).

The reception is held at my cousin Stephen's hotel. ('Fantastic,' he said, in his usual deep, almost monotone voice when I asked him weeks ago if it was available. 'And it goes without saying, Elise, that you will get the "family" rate, although in your case that's actually more expensive than the regular rate.') Anne and Angela cry during my speech. Many people laugh during it, too. ('There are things Evan will never do, and we have to be realistic … [pause for effect] … He will never be the first black president.')

When it is time to feed Evan I realise I have everything I need except the pole that raises the bag of liquid food high enough to allow gravity to suck it down into the tube and then into the peg inserted into the button in his abdomen. Anne and her partner Richard, Neil B and Violet spring into action and form a human conveyor line. Each holds something – a piece of tubing, the vent circuit (to keep it out of the way), the feeding pump – and they take it in turns to hold the bag up high. It's a team effort.

Later, I take Evan back to the hospital, get him into his pyjamas and tuck him into bed with a kiss and a cuddle. Then I return to the hotel for a night of laughter, surrounded by many of the most important people in my life.

4 April 2013

Sergeant Accomando finally replies to my multiple attempts to contact him. He writes that the case has not reached the level of probable cause to make an arrest. I reply, reminding him that we have the expert report of Dr Kathryn Grimm, which says that, given the timing and the severity of the injuries, Norma must have been the person responsible. I end that email with, 'Pardon my frankness, but it sounds to me like you are letting her walk away.'

This at least spurs an immediate response from him. He goes on a bit about how he isn't pleased about all the inconsistencies of her statements, and then says, 'The police department has exhausted all leads at this time.' He ends with a lecture on how Norma's arrest won't help Evan; only God can do that.

I'm not sure what annoys me more. I have always known that a conviction won't help Evan, and I have always understood that it wouldn't help me either. And I most certainly don't need a police officer to talk about God with me (what happened to the separation of Church and State?). But I have always trusted that the authorities would do what they needed to do without having to involve me. These last few months I have tried to stay on top of those authorities so that I can be satisfied they did do what they had to do, whether that resulted in an arrest or a conviction or not. But now I am being patronised by a police officer who hasn't explored too many leads at all, but is sick of hearing from me and now says all the leads are exhausted?

I follow up with several more emails over several days but don't hear anything else from Sergeant Accomando. I even ask him to give me the District Attorney's details, but still nothing in response. Eventually I call the Child Abuse Division and tell them I want to file a complaint against Accomando. I don't get to do that because instead I am promised – and receive – an email from an Inspector Mike Keenan.

Inspector Keenan addresses me as 'Mr Schwarz' and then says 'Sorry for your loss'. It isn't too good a start. Later, though, we have a long conversation on the phone and I feel a bit better. He says he is the new head of the department and that he is making Evan's case a priority. We shall see. He also says that Norma was originally interviewed back in March 2012 but had requested a lawyer and they didn't get to ask any questions after that. I didn't know that until now.

I send Inspector Keenan everything I have, the timeline with exhibits, the letters I wrote, everything. That should give him some night-time reading for a while.

7 April 2013

It dawned on me recently that I don't have any paperwork from the court (and none from ACS, of course) to indicate the family court case is over, so I email Randi and ask her to get me a copy of the judgement against Norma. Randi asks Lubin, who emails it to her. When she forwards it to me, she adds a note to tell me that the wording of the judgement against Norma is ambiguous. I take a look and, sure enough, although the caption no longer bears my name and the document clearly applies only to Norma, it refers to her in a couple of places as the 'Respondent Mother'.

I am livid. Randi steps in once again and tells me she will get Lubin to have it fixed (as Randi's role ended when the case against me was dropped, she doesn't have a direct route to the judge any more).

Lubin writes back, 'The clerk shouldn't have used the word "mother", but since the case is already over, I wouldn't worry about it.'

I nearly have a fit at his casualness. Instead, I sit down and write a letter to the judge.

Re: In the Matter of Evan Schwarz v Norma Leonce
Docket # NA 12099-12
CPS 6657001

Dear Judge Richardson:

As you may recall, I am the mother of Evan Schwarz, the minor in the above-referenced case. Although an action was commenced against me initially, you dismissed it (on the grounds of reliance on expert evidence) on September 13, 2012.

As you will be reminded by the attached Order of Fact Finding and Disposition, Norma Leonce, Evan's former babysitter, was found guilty of child abuse and certain conditions were imposed on her.

I just received a copy of this document two days ago. I was very disturbed to read that Leonce had been referred to as the 'Respondent Mother' (See page 2, 'Order of Disposition –highlighted). This is, of course, a typo, and should read simply 'Respondent', since Leonce is not related to Evan. However, it creates confusion to any reader: without scrutiny the implication is that I, as the mother, am the one receiving conditions. This causes me great consternation. I am also concerned that the judgment itself has no real effect on Leonce due to this error.

I asked my former attorney, Randi L. Karmel, Esq., to informally take the matter up with ACS, since it is their case, and to ask that they ensure the issue is corrected. The response Ms Karmel received from Jesse Lubin, Esq. was 'The clerk shouldn't have used the word "mother", but since the case is already over, I wouldn't worry about it.'

I find this response to be as concerning as it is illuminating. Jesse Lubin, Esq., and his organisation brought an action against me with total disregard to the facts (as collected by their investigators). He failed to bring any action against

Leonce for three months, allowing her to continue to work with infants during that time. Now, having been told that the judgment they did obtain against Leonce is fundamentally flawed, he does not feel the need to move the Court to correct it.

It is my personal opinion that this represents a repeatedly cavalier attitude of a member of the New York bar, and that it is quite reprehensible, especially given the power that I believe he wields. It is incredible to me that my own child was wrongly removed from my custody on the request of this attorney and his organisation, and yet I can see no concern shown when the real offender is not properly accounted for in the judgment against her.

I am also left to wonder why, once again, I have to do ACS' footwork for them.

Given the massive financial outlay ACS' wrongful action against me caused me to incur (not to mention the extreme emotional distress they inflicted on me in an already horrific time) I am unable to ask Ms Karmel to represent me further, and hence this *amicus* letter to the Court.

Please ensure the judgment is corrected accordingly. I would very much appreciate it if you could send me a corrected version.

Yours truly,

Elise Schwarz

A few days later, Randi, who hasn't seen my letter, forwards me an email she has received from Lubin. He has copied it to his supervisors at ACS.

> Hi Randi,
>
> In retrospect I should not have minimised the fact that the Order was incorrect and I apologise. I did not mean to minimise this case, what Ms Schwarz went through as a result of it, or what she continues to go through with her son's condition. I have spoken to Judge Richardson and the Order is being corrected and will be sent to Ms Schwarz. Please let her know that I am sorry.

Oh, what sweet success – an apology (of sorts) from Lubin, and the knowledge that he has been roasted over Judge Richardson's coals. It's probably the only satisfaction I will ever get for what ACS did to me in my darkest hours, but I've learnt to take my victories where I find them these days.

8 April 2013

I spend some time every day getting Evan down on the mat on the floor of the ward, next to his bed. I roll him from side to side. He grunts in complaint, and it's not graceful. But I'm told it's good for him.

Since the christening (my first time taking Evan out without a nurse) I've been taking him outside on my own every few days. It takes about forty-five minutes to get everything ready (the vent positioned properly on his pushchair; the pulse-ox and the suction units arranged; Evan dressed in suitable clothes), which is always longer than the amount of time I take him outside for. I don't have a great deal of confidence yet. I'm still put off by people staring (even though there are lots of sick children around), and it's been quite cold and windy outside recently, which makes me worry whether Evan is comfortable. This is especially so given the fact that he still can't blink. I've invested in a pair of children's sunglasses for him, but it still worries me. Also, the hospital is built on a hill with surprisingly few disabled ramps from the pavement to the road. His buggy is extremely heavy with all his equipment (and him) I have an image I will trip on the kerb and Evan will go hurtling down Argyle Street.

One of the nurses asks if she can come with us on our walk today: the ward is quiet and she is bored. I am glad of the company. Without a word, she has us down the hill, across two busy streets and up the disabled ramp into the Glasgow Art Gallery and Museum, a ten-minute walk away. It's a bit of a revelation. The place is bustling with children on their Easter holiday outings. No one stares at Evan. It gives me a glimpse of future possibilities for outings we can do alone.

9 April 2013

There is a sensory room two floors above our ward. It's a small room with blackout blinds on the windows and cushions on the floor. There are various lights and mirrors that can be adjusted to create any kind of kaleidoscopic experience you like. Evan and I go up there a couple of times a week and lie on the cushions, side by side, staring at the images of light reflected on the ceiling. It's bliss just to be able to talk to him without feeling self-conscious about others hearing, and without being distracted or interrupted. I tell him we'll be home soon; that one day he will be able to run around in Granny's garden; that we'll get a dog, and maybe even a camper van and go off on holiday around Scotland.

When we get back from the sensory room today, PT comes over and compliments me on Evan's progress.

'It's a testament to all the work you are doing with him that he's making these improvements.'

She seems very genuine. I am really quite confused at the compliment, though, because I'm not sure anyone but me can see him improving. And really all he is doing is moving a tiny bit, every now and then. Mind you, it's typically Scottish to not be able to accept a compliment, so perhaps I have just re-acclimatised myself to being here.

26 April 2013

Since the christening, my cousin Stephen has really become interested in raising money for Yorkhill. We raised a tidy amount for it that day just by raffling off some cheap Easter eggs. Stephen has a friend who has a hotel on the other side of the city and who sent me along to a charity night they were having last night. It was some kind of 'sportsmen's' event.

When I got there, there were about a thousand guys in suits and ten women, including me. There was an MC who is apparently a well-known food critic and football pundit (I hadn't heard of him). Stephen's friend starts the proceedings off by standing up and telling everyone about the charities the dinner is in aid of. He speaks at length about the Alzheimer's charity that he is promoting, and about how his mother has Alzheimer's. Then he introduces me, and I get up and speak about Evan's journey, how he almost died, the move from New York to Glasgow, and how great Yorkhill is for both of us.

Once I sit down (to polite applause), the MC stands up. I suppose you could describe him as very typically Glaswegian.

'Jesus Christ,' he begins, 'I need a bloody violin after all of that!'

Then he launches into his own raucous and very blue monologue, which is met with peals of laughter. At the end, he gives a push for the charities again, then adds, 'Where's that lassie from New York?'

I raise my hand, reluctantly.

'Aye, you! How do you like slumming it here in Glasgow

then, eh? Away back to New York and stop making us all feel bad about ourselves.'

It is truly hilarious and very embarrassing but by the end of the night we have raised a very impressive sum for Yorkhill, so it is worth it.

3 May 2013

Evan's eyes continue to be a source of concern. Not having a blink reflex is a serious issue, as is the fact that he can't close them over completely when he sleeps. The right eye has improved a bit, but the left one still shows a large sliver of blue, which the air gets to. It means the scratch to the cornea has not been able to heal completely. I'm told it's not infected, but that it's not getting any better. The eye doctor called me a few days ago and told me the next step is to give him a Botox injection into each eyelid. He says we have exhausted all other options and it's the only solution: Botox will paralyse the muscle and the lid will close. If we do that, it will take about three months for the Botox to wear off, and only then will he be able to open his eyes again.

I really hate that idea.

The eye doctor has an appointment with us today. He says he will come prepared to give the injection, but will first examine Evan's eyes (amazingly, he hasn't ever seen Evan – he is only basing his thoughts on the referring doctor's notes). Unluckily for his medical assistant, however, she has missed part of the plan, and walks into our ward a few minutes ahead of the eye doctor.

'I'm here to give Evan his Botox,' she smiles.

In her hand are two filled syringes with needles attached.

'Is that the Botox?' I ask.

'Yes,' she replies.

This sets me off. It's one thing to find myself faced with a quandary – shut the eyes for the long-term solution, or keep the sight for the short-term. It's quite another to be rushed too many steps ahead like this so I let her know I have heightened emotions about the issue.

When the eye doctor shows up he is quite surprised to find his assistant looking a bit upset, and the mother of his patient with steam coming from her ears. He examines Evan, realises his eyes aren't quite as bad as he had thought, and goes with my suggestion that we increase the eye-care treatment (eye drops and ointment), cover the left eye with a plaster to allow intensive healing, and revisit the issue in another week.

When they have both left a nurse comes over to us. I worry briefly that she will think I have gone too far this time.

'Quite right,' she says. 'You handled that well.'

Then she sets about giving instructions for every nurse to abide by the following week.

'We want to win this,' she tells me, as she writes in Evan's medical notes.

All of this coincides with me losing my phone. I never lose things and this is really annoying as it has all my photographs of Evan since we arrived in Scotland on it. I debate with myself whether to pray for it to be found. These days I reserve every single one of my prayers for Evan's full recovery, and refuse to pray for anything else but I reason that the photos of Evan really are for his sake as well. I also think that my prayers to God probably sound a bit like white noise to Him at this stage. I decide it is acceptable to vary them a bit and pray for my phone to be found.

However, as I sit holding Evan I shoot God another one: 'Dear God, keep the phone, save the eyes!'

10 May 2013

It's Connie Connolly's birthday. My beloved childhood babysitter would be 104 years old if she were still alive (and she is the only grown-up female I have ever met who treated every passing birthday as another feather in her cap). I usually get a treat for myself on this day, but instead I walk over to Byres Road in the West End to a boutique children's shop and buy Evan a pair of old-fashioned looking blue and white pyjamas.

Connie would have loved them – she would have warmed them at the fire before putting them on him.

13 May 2013

Jeez, I got my 'metabolic age' checked out today! It is fifty-nine. I'm only forty-two!!!!

Back in Glasgow

My furniture arrived today, a good two months later than the estimated arrival date, and at a whopping fifty per cent more expense than it was estimated at. Still, I'm glad I have it. In all this change, it's a physical reminder of a time when we were truly happy.

I've spent the last few weeks clearing out the attic in my mum's house, scrubbing the walls, and sanding and varnishing the floorboards. Now my furniture is in there it's like a little apartment. I need to feel I've got my own space.

It's a nice space. The ceiling is lower than in the other rooms of the house (about eight foot high at best) and slants with the roof. The room wraps around its own stairwell, and the walls of that are white painted oak panels. The walls inside the attic are wooden and varnished. It's a kind of 'Hamptons beach house' meets 'cabin in the woods' effect. I always found it to be very creepy as a child, but actually, if you put the right pieces of furniture in the right places and light it properly, it's the most interesting room in the house.

I reacquaint myself with my things, and I spend a lot of time going through boxes I would have thrown away, had I had time to do so before we left. In one I find my diary from January 2012. On the first page it reads:

'Resolutions: lose weight, attend baby classes with Evan, try to learn a language (again), try to stop hugging people as much'. (I am an over-hugger.)

For once I have an excuse for not fulfilling this list.

16 May 2013

The eye doctor is very impressed with the improvement in Evan's eyes during these past few weeks and isn't considering Botox any more. Hurrah! And I still haven't found my phone so I guess the prayer worked. I did, however, find a way to access the lost photos via my computer, so God seems to be in a generous mood these days.

Then I have a conversation with Dr Davies. He says he is reluctant to make any changes to the vent. I know where he is going with this so I pre-empt him to get it over with.

'You're saying this because you don't think he can get off the vent.'

'No, I don't,' he says, shaking his head kindly but firmly.

'Well, I disagree with you on that, because I've seen him taking breaths every now and then. Not often, and not consistently, but they happen.'

He doesn't try and contradict me, which is nice. Maybe I can get him to experiment a bit.

Funnily enough, this is a conversation I might not have been able to have were it not for the fact that we have just won the Botox War. It has given me a confidence that I haven't enjoyed to date. Evan's eye is not as bad as they initially thought. That means other things might be better than predicted too.

17 May 2013

Every evening I call the ward around 8.45pm. It is almost

always the same conversation ('Yes, he's fine, fast asleep'). I always wish there was more to be said. Sometimes, right after I hang up, I feel disappointed that I won't have another reason to contact him/the ward until the morning. Tonight, though, the nurse tells me Evan is looking quite blotchy and a bit unsettled. I say I will be right there. I know there isn't anything seriously wrong. Because he can't cry out or even screw up his face, blotchiness is Evan's way of communicating unhappiness. If something is really wrong, his heart rate will shoot up or he will desat.

As there is no actual emergency, it's a pleasure to be driving towards the hospital, knowing my being with him will help him. He's a bit more settled by the time I get there, but he is also taking a few of his big gulping breaths, which is always a pleasure to see. I sit with him for an hour or so, until he is fully relaxed and sound asleep. Then I go home, happy, knowing he is happier, too.

13 May 2013

Today is an amazing day. I wake up still feeling good about seeing Evan last night and go to the hospital at my usual time in the morning. When I get there I sit with him on my lap as usual, but then I realise there is something a little different about how he feels. I lift him up, turn him around and sit him on the edge of his bed, still supporting him at his armpits. Sure enough, there it is.

Evan is holding his own head up.

It feels like magic. Or at least a start. And we've needed a start for a long time. I let it happen a few more times before I tell one of the nurses. She is impressed, but I get the impression she can't remember if this is something he could do before or not — she sees a lot of different babies in here.

Anyway, I have been high as a kite all day. I had plans to go out tonight to a friend's house for a barbecue, but I just can't think of having a conversation with anyone about anything other than Evan holding his head up. Nor do I want alcohol to numb the joy I'm feeling. So I cancel. I buy a tin of blue paint on the way home and then set about painting the room that will be Evan's when he comes home.

19 May 2013

I wake up exhausted after a very light sleep, but still excited about the head holding. Then I get into a real downer, thinking about the possibility that he might not do it again today — perhaps it was just a one-off.

I manage to get myself into a foul mood by the time I walk into the ward this morning, but there is no need. As soon as I put Evan on my lap, he sits with a straight back and his head balancing properly on his neck. He can't hold it up indefinitely — there comes a point where it gets too much for him and it just flops forward. I try and catch his forehead with my lips when he does this, cushioning him with a nice soft kiss.

He won't get any prizes for deportment right now, but we can work on the finer points over time. It just fills me with hope. And it opens up so many possibilities, most of which involve high chairs.

Back home, Mum and I celebrate with chocolate profiteroles.

30 May 2013

Chatting with Violet on the phone today, I tell her about Evan's head and how things just feel so much better.

'And I haven't had to rely on Ativan for such a long time. I only take it...'

'Recreationally?' she butts in.

Yes, she is right. I have still been taking the occasional Ativan and it's not because I need to. My anxiety levels are way down. I tell myself I take it when I want to sleep, but the reality is I like the way it makes me feel far more than is healthy. I find the bottle and flush the remaining pills down the toilet.

31 May 2013

I take Evan down to the cafeteria on the first floor today. We go down there every now and then. It's my way of letting the ward know I'm happy to take him out, I'm independent, we are doing just fine on our own, etc., etc. It's also my way of avoiding the stress of taking him out for a walk outside the hospital.

After a quick scone and cup of tea I get up and start pushing Evan towards the door. A man walks in front of us. I'd seen him get up to leave and had planned our exit at the same time, as it's always handy to get someone to hold open the door into the corridor so I can push the buggy through with both hands. He has a tray of food in his hands, though, and as soon as he is through the door, he lets it swing behind him and I have to negotiate it by myself after all. This is what leads me to keep looking at him when we finally get into the corridor. As he walks in front, he passes the men's bathroom. Then he stops and walks back, pushes the door to the bathroom open with his back, and (because the door closes very slowly) I see him place his tray of food on top of the bin in the bathroom while he leaves it to do what he has gone in there to do. As I continue our walk towards the lifts, I think how disgusting that is.

The lift takes a long time to come, and by the time it does, the man with the tray has caught up with us. We all get in the lift. After a few moments, another man in the lift turns to the man with the tray and says, 'That smells delicious.'

'It's my wife's,' he replies.

2 June 2013

I'm waiting for my mood to lighten.

I am so sick of being in hospital. Yes, it is miles better than life at Blythedale – it is infinitely less boring – but there is no privacy (in Blythedale there was often too much privacy). I am aerating negativity vibes to try and stop anyone and everyone from talking to us. I just want to be with Evan. I don't want anyone to interrupt our time together so they can tell me about the chips they had last night or how many buses it takes them to get to work.

It doesn't work, though. I sit and listen as a nurse (not a regular) tells the mother of the baby next to Evan what an improvement she sees in him, how he is so clever – oh, look at what he can do. Then she turns to me and says, 'Evan is… getting so big!'

Yes, it does hurt to hear platitudes and compliments bestowed on other people's children and not on my own. And yes, I do know how petty and childish that makes me sound.

5 June 2013

We have a 'progress meeting' today. The vent services coordinator, two nurses, two doctors and me all meet in a small, windowless room in the basement on the other side of the hospital.

Dr Davies explains that because Evan has been stable for a long time now we can start to think about getting him home. He says that even though, officially, we have been waiting for carers to become available, he would not have discharged Evan until now (almost six months in) anyway, because of the medical issues Evan has had. This is in marked contrast to the attitude at Blythedale, where they would have discharged him very early on, regardless of stability, if it hadn't been for the ACS case.

Then the vent services coordinator explains that, as has been the case all along, there still aren't any carers available to look after him at home, and there probably won't be any until September.

I didn't think we would have quite so long to wait. We are

number two on the list now, as the first two babies have managed to get off their vents and have gone home. The third (now the first) looks like he's about to do the same. If he does, that will bring us to the top of the list. But there isn't much to do other than wait.

It is a good conversation with Dr Davies, though. I tell him again that I disagree with his prognosis that Evan will never be able to breathe. Then I ask him if, assuming just for a second that I am right and he is wrong, whether any detriments to Evan's breathing development are taking place because we aren't attempting to wean him off it right now. Dr Davies says that no, there will be no difference made to the autonomic process if it is going to come back. He also says if Evan does show signs of improvement in his breathing then he will take the appropriate action, adding, 'I'm not closed to the possibility.' Knowing there is still the slightest possibility of Evan being able to breathe again when he is ready feels like a half-step up.

20 June 2013

I post a photograph of Evan on Facebook today. His eyes are wide open and bright. They can't really move, and he still can't blink, but there is more light showing than before. People have started commenting on how he has my eyes – they used to say that all the time. I realise now how much I have missed hearing that.

Back in Glasgow

28 June 2013

I have started taking Evan home for a few hours every few days. After the Progress Meeting I realised that I had to step up to the plate if I wanted him to come home for good.

At first I was terrified. I only did it on days when Margaret was there, and I could plant myself and Evan on the couch and refuse to move – not even to go to the bathroom – for an hour or so and then call a taxi to take us back to the hospital. After a week or two though, I became gradually more comfortable. Now I can even leave him alone for long enough to make myself a cup of tea – although I have a video camera on him then and I take the monitor into the kitchen with me so I can check on his face and his pulse-ox while I am away from him.

It's been liberating, though, getting him out of the hospital. In fact, the more I do it, the less I can stand the days when we have to stay in the hospital. I would take him home every single day if I could, but I have to put him in a hackney cab (I can't drive and take care of his ventilation needs at the same time) and that really gets expensive.

I've started to know far more about Glasgow hackney drivers than I ever did before. For one thing, they have a pride in their job that would make a New York cab driver turn off his meter and stare. Glasgow hackney drivers are really more like New York limo or town car drivers. They are almost always courteous, smartly dressed and know where they're going. More often than not they will strike up a conversation with you. One driver told me in great detail that he had just had the best boiled-egg-on-toast sandwich ever. 'You know how sometimes you just boil it to perfection? Well, this was like that. And I sliced it perfectly so it reached the edges of the slice of bread without overlapping. It was a Hovis loaf too, brown. I don't think I'll ever make a better one.'

They tell me they are a gossipy lot. They hang out at taxi ranks and chat like fishwives. They have names for some of their colleagues too. The 'Wing' is missing his right arm. 'Heart Beat' has had four heart attacks. 'Butter Bean... nobody likes butterbeans, do they?' I'm not sure I've ever been picked up by any of these characters. I only know our drivers by the condition of their ramps that I use to wheel Evan's chair into the cab. One ramp is missing one of two pivots that secure it to the cab floor. Another ramp bends inwards instead of sloping in a straight line. 'It's not broken, it's just flexible,' that driver told me.

One day I came out and the taxi driver didn't have his ramp out because he thought Evan's pushchair was just a regular buggy. When he saw all the wires and the vent he quickly went to fetch it from the back of his taxi. 'Sorry, love,' he said to me. 'That's not what I was expecting.'

'Me neither,' I replied.

He was too polite to laugh.

Another time I had to take a taxi to the hospital in the morning because I had a flat tyre on Mum's car. I told the driver about it. He got quite annoyed at me for not knowing how to change a tyre. 'You're just like my wife,' he said. Then we arranged a time for him to collect me from the hospital in the evening. He showed up, drove me home and changed my tyre for me. He showed me what he was doing and how. 'Now you'll know for next time,' he said. (Next time I'll just give him a call, I think to myself.)

1 July 2013

I decide to have a late start today, possibly to go into town, or for lunch, before heading up to the hospital later in the afternoon. I just really need some time away from the ward. Around 11am, though, a man comes to the door. He calls himself a tree surgeon and he has a Highland accent.

'Sorry to say,' he lilts, 'but that's an awful mess that's been made of that holly tree.'

He gets his two buddies to come over and they take a look, hoisting one of them up so he stands on the stump at the top.

'Aye, it's a right mess. It's been cut too low, and it hasn't been treated. It's drying up. To be honest, I don't think it's going to live through the next winter.'

They give it a treatment and lop some more dead branches off it. Once they are done, I ask them what the chances are of it living.

'We'll pray,' says the one who has seen the worst of it.

I want to say, 'If you're praying, can you forget the tree and just focus on Evan?'

Once they have gone I feel utterly sick and tired of being upset over the tree once again. I don't want to be preoccupied by it when I have so much else to worry about, but I just can't seem to help it.

I Believe in Evan

7 July 2013

I send another email to Inspector Keenan, asking for an update. I've emailed him every few weeks since he took over Evan's case. He always has something to say, but never convinces me that there is anything going on at all. It feels like I'm being Accomando-ed again.

I cheer up when I arrive at the ward, though: Evan is sitting up in his buggy. He looks great. His eyes are clear and bright. I call out to him and he turns his head towards me. Later, when I am holding him, his head flips forward, but this time he lifts it back up all on his own.

13 July 2013

Evan's eyes have such a look of sadness in them today. This is big news: he can show some emotion through his eyes. So far I've had to rely on the pulse-ox to see what his heart rate is doing. That and the level of blotchiness on his face have been my only real measure of my boy's mood. After a good long cuddle with me the sadness leaves them.

25 July 2013

I feel quite ashamed. Evan got a new chair today. I asked for his seat to be adjusted so that he faces me, instead of facing outwards where I can't see him. I said it was because I want to see him and for him to see me. That's seventy-five per cent right. But it's also partly motivated by my not wanting adults to stare at him (kids are fine, they're not usually judgemental).

26 July 2013

Inspector Keenan emails me to say they are in the process of interviewing some of the witnesses, including Norma's past employers. He says that Norma will be re-interviewed at some point but not yet.

29 July 2013

Anne and Pauline are staying in Glasgow for their summer holidays, along with their partners and Pauline's two gorgeous little girls. We've been having a truly lovely time. Pauline has taken up golf and makes all of us go out to the pitch and putt at Queen's Park frequently so she can try and beat us (when she can't, she cheats). We've been having evenings outside in Mum's garden, with the chimenea burning the wood from the big tree (it's been lying in neat piles at the bottom of the garden since it fell down, nineteen months ago) and the barbecue going. It's been the most glorious summer, actually. We have had day after day of soaring heat and sunshine.

I bring Evan home for a visit. I'm not sure why, but I become really teary. I think it is (in part) because today's taxi driver asks me question after question about Evan. I often get asked what happened to Evan and I always say something like, 'He had a brain haemorrhage after a bad seizure.' Today's driver keeps asking more and more questions ('What caused the seizure?'

'Will he get better?'). He has already gone too far before I remember I can tell him I don't want to talk about it.

By the time I get home I am feeling pretty low. Once I get Evan in the house, there is such joviality and happiness all round as everyone gets ready to go out and enjoy more sunshine. I have to fight hard to stop the tears from starting. They ask me if I want to come, but I say no, Evan and I will sit on the couch and keep Mum company. When they have gone, I can't hold it in any more. I sob and sob. Mum has no idea why – and neither do I, really. I suppose it's just another realisation that Evan and I can't be part of the fun in the way that we should be.

I cry so much that I suddenly feel Evan shift in my arms. He throws his head backwards and looks at me. He must wonder what I am doing. His head falls forward but he manages to throw it back one more time to take another look. It is heart-warming. I keep crying, though.

1 August 2013

There is very limited activity in the hospital. The physiotherapist still comes by once a week and shows me new stretches for Evan, and then I do them as often as I can with him. A music teacher comes to the ward once a week and has a music class in the playroom across from Evan's room. Any child can attend, whether sick or just visiting. The teacher is wonderful. She sings in a high voice and gives each child a rattle or a drum to make noises with. Sometimes there are as many as twelve little babies in the class, sitting on a parent or nurse's knee, rattling away.

She brings a huge amount of positivity with her and for the rest of the day us parents walk around saying hi to each other and smiling about the session.

Apart from that, though, there isn't much stimulation for Evan at all. I was getting increasingly impatient waiting for another week to roll around until we could get our music class again, so a few weeks ago I talked to the physiotherapist and asked her to point us in the direction of other therapies or play groups. She told me about Sense Scotland, which is a charity for people of all ages who have sensory impairments.

I contacted Sense and arranged a meeting with one of its therapists, Rachael, who then came and visited Evan and me in Yorkhill. I was amazed at how easily she sang out little songs to Evan, even though there were at least fifteen nurses and therapists watching. I felt quite overwhelmed by the interest from everyone, but Rachael took it all in her stride. Before she left, she invited us to come to the Sense facility, known as TouchBase, and check it out for myself.

TouchBase is an eye opener. It's housed in a big building in Kinning Park, just across the river from Yorkhill. The space has lots of natural light. There is a large cafeteria area as you walk in, which is very welcoming, and is open to the public too. There are people from all age groups there, being helped by their individual therapists. Some seem to have almost no ability to function independently at all. Others can clearly do a lot for themselves. There are some young men in wheelchairs, wearing crash helmets. Some teenagers call out loudly and suddenly at times, but everyone there seems used to that. There are staff members everywhere, and many of the people have one-on-one care. The overall atmosphere is extremely happy.

The first time we go to TouchBase the lady at the cash register of the cafeteria asks me all about Evan. The next time we go, she recognises us and calls her colleague over to meet him.

'This wee boy can sleep with his eyes open,' she boasts.

I feel huge pride for Evan at that.

We've now had several art classes at Sense and each time I can see something in Evan that I haven't seen before. The teacher, Mhàiri, gets Evan and I to sit astride a music log, and then, still sitting, we start swaying backwards and forwards and round and round with Evan. We make up our own sounds, so he can associate each movement. 'Whoooop' for a circular twist in one direction and then 'whiiiirlll' when we come around the other way. Evan's eyes become really big. A few times he starts vocalising. He has a real reaction to the stimulation – certainly the most I've seen from him so far.

Another teacher, Susanne, has been coming to the house once a week – Evan and I meet her there. She is part of the 'Parent Enabler Project', which is designed to give parents like me ideas of how to get the most from our children. She does all sorts of things, but the most significant thing she has brought to us so far is a resonance board. It's basically just a piece of plywood – about 3 feet by 4 feet – set on little legs, raising it about an inch off the ground. The idea is that Evan lies on it, and then any sound made by his movement 'resonates' and he can hear it much louder. Depending on exactly how loud the noise is he might even feel its vibrations through the board. That might encourage him to make the movement again. Within a couple of sessions of trying the resonance board we started to see Evan's legs try very hard to move. At first it is barely perceptible. Gradually, though, both legs start to twitch, independently of each other, and his face looks tense, as if he is trying his very best.

We've had a few more sessions since that first breakthrough, and each time Evan has shown the same kind of movement. Every time I walk Susanne to the front door, we beam about how good a session we have had.

3 August 2013

I've known for a few weeks now that I'm not grieving any more. The baby I have mourned for would be gone by now anyway. I'm able to look at photographs of Evan as a healthy baby again. I can enjoy videos of him laughing, yawning, sleeping. I can remember our walks through Central Park with happiness now.

Of course, he's not the toddler I was expecting. He can't walk or talk, or move or breathe. Often I feel deep sadness at that, though I've somehow learnt to live with it. It's not the same grinding feeling of grieving, though. That has gone.

15 August 2013

Everything is now in place for Evan to come home. We just have to wait for his new bed (the same type as he has in the hospital) to be delivered to the house.

I can't wait. I've been painting everything that is static in the house. Evan's room couldn't be more ready. The walls are a perfect baby blue. The curtains are blue, with a faint red stripe. The bookshelves have been put together, and the thousands of cuddly toys given to Evan over these past two years are displayed to look as though they are eagerly anticipating his return.

I know it's going to be great, but I also know it's going to be a big change for me. When Evan comes home I won't be able to leave the house much. At least one carer will be with him eighteen hours a day (10pm until 4pm), but there has to be a 'responsible second person' around at all times too. We will go to TouchBase as much as we can, and we can go for walks, if the rain stays off.

Knowing how life is about to change once again, I am forced to concede this would all be easier if I had another half. If I ever had motivation to navigate the pain that comes with a relationship again, now would be that time – and at my most undesirable moment. My online profile would have to read, 'Seeks true love and ventilator proficiency. Must like the elderly too.'

23 August 2013

I am told that the bed is coming next Thursday. I get so excited that I leave Evan early to get things ready. I'm not sure what 'things' I feel are not yet ready, but as I spin my wheels stuck in traffic, on the way home I take a detour to a furniture place and order new flooring for the kitchen and bathroom. Then I buy some paint for two more rooms, along with brushes and rollers. I get home, now very high on the scale of overexcitable, and tell my mum everything that has happened to me in the previous two hours. She, needless to say, feels overwhelmed and anxious about the whole thing, which brings me crashing down. I take a three-hour nap on the couch and wake up in the dark with the TV on and the curtains still open. I'll take the paint back tomorrow. The flooring is still a good idea, though (and I've already paid to have someone other than me take care of installing it).

24 August 2013

An email war with Inspector Keenan has left me feeling bruised and annoyed. I have emailed him a few times over the last three weeks and received no reply, so last night I reached the end of my rope and emailed him to tell him that in the five months since he has taken over, very little has been done and now he won't even communicate with me. He emails back a few lame excuses and I challenge him on each one. (I also add 'and my name is Elise, not Elsie' – he's been addressing me as that since the beginning). This morning he sends a short and snippy reply that ends with 'You obviously don't think I know how to run an investigation.' I hold back on replying, 'Well, now you come to mention it…' and instead write, 'Who do you think you are? My son can't blink, never mind breathe or move.'

He replies quickly with an apology, and finally gives me the District Attorney's details (I've been asking for that since last October – why the big secret?).

29 August 2013

Talking to some of the nurses on the ward today, holding Evan in my lap, laughing at something light-heartedly, my phone rings. It's a district attorney from the Manhattan DA's office. He explains that a lot of investigation has already been done on the case and that meetings are held every couple of months or so. I don't really believe him but that's what he says. Then he tells me he doesn't think he can gather enough of a case against Norma.

'The problem is, although some doctors will say the time of onset in a case as serious as Evan's has to have been right before the cardiac arrest, there are plenty of SBS expert medics who will say that it's not possible to tell when it happened, more than in a 24-hour period.'

I try to argue with him. I begin by telling him to bring his best case and let Norma figure out if she can get an expert to refute it. Somewhere in the middle of the conversation I realise I have to back off. I'm starting to go down a road of seeking vengeance, no matter what. I ceded responsibility for finding justice to the NYPD and the DA's office in the very early days, and this has always been the wisest thing to do. But here I am, now insisting it's all about winning against Norma – not about finding out the truth – and not about being rational and reasoned so as to avoid a miscarriage of justice. I let the conversation conclude. The DA ends by telling me that they will interview Norma anyway, to see if she says anything about what happened. I tell him that would be very meaningful to me.

Later, he sends me an email with his details.

'I'm very sorry to have had to give you that news by telephone,' the email reads. By this time I have settled down again. I want to write this to him: 'I have never needed Norma to go to jail. I have always deferred to the authorities as to what would happen to her. My role, as far as I can see, is to be peaceful and calm and loving towards Evan. Your role is to pursue justice for him. It has only been important to me to ensure that you do not neglect to do that.'

But I don't send him any reply at all. Just as it is not for me to push the issue, it is equally not for me to give him the green light to relax his efforts.

Do I need to know what Norma did to Evan, though? In my heart, I still don't think what she did (whatever she did) was done maliciously. I could be wrong about that, so maybe I don't want/need to know the truth after all. Either way, Norma going to prison will not help Evan. Norma going to prison if she doesn't deserve to would be a travesty. She can't work with children any more, and she also has to live with herself, even if there are no further repercussions.

I wish we could employ a 'Truth and Reconciliation Commission' as they did in post-apartheid South Africa. Victims got to tell their aggressors what they had been through at their hands. If the aggressor was truthful, and could show that he had only been operating under governmental orders, he was given an amnesty. There were actually very few of these amnesties handed out, and probably a lot of 'truth' was withheld by the guilty trying to qualify for them. But apparently it did do a lot of good for a lot of South Africans: it helped the nation heal and move forward.

However, even if it were a perfect system, there isn't any vehicle for it in the New York criminal justice system. There is no way a DA would waive his or her right to prosecute just because Norma promised to tell the truth. If she confesses to hurting Evan, she has to be punished for it. So there isn't any motivation at all for her to say what happened to Evan.

My thoughts go round and round in circles, trying to figure out a way to settle myself. After a while I think about what I would say to Norma if we were allowed our own 'Truth and Reconciliation Commission'. And, as I learnt to do over and over again in my therapy sessions just south of Union Square, I write her a letter, with no intention of sending it.

When I am finished I know I am also finished with Norma, and with thinking about whatever she did or didn't do.

Evan, my son, let's go home.

His room is ready. He will sleep in there at night-time. During the day, he will go into the front bedroom. It has beautiful bay windows and is a lot lighter than his bedroom. The two silver birches are to be thanked for falling down and letting all that light in (and I will try to ignore the stump of the holly tree that is clearly visible at the side).

The walls in the front bedroom are peach-coloured, so he can know the front room is a different place from the room he sleeps in (which is blue). There's a lot more space, too (his equipment has made his bedroom feel very claustrophobic). In the evening, when there is no carer, he will come downstairs and sit with Mum and me in the front room, which is mostly decorated in cream colours and (for now, anyway) receives beautiful evening sunshine. Then, when the night carer comes in at 10pm, we will carry him (and all his equipment) back to his bedroom upstairs.

Part Six

At Home

31 August 2013

Evan spends his first night at home. This is his 'practice night'.
One of his carers meets us at the house and almost as soon as
we get inside, Evan's trachy pops right out of his stoma. Within
seconds, with the carer's help, I have replaced it with a new one
and everything is fine again. Mum watches all of this happen
from her seat on the couch. She is quite shocked. Poor Mum.
I have a strong track record of dropping her in at the deep
end of my life over things that I myself have been given a long
time to get used to first ('I'm gay!' 'I'm pregnant!' And now,
'Emergency tube change!').

The practice night goes well. Evan appears very comfortable

in his new bed. The carer sits in a chair in his room all night. I sleep lightly, if at all, in the bedroom next door. The carer leaves us this morning at 8am, as planned. Evan and I have a luxurious few hours lying on the couch together, me telling him all our plans, him looking quite keen to hear them, I'd say.

Later, we go for a walk in Newlands Park, which is only five minutes from home. The sunshine is bright and crisp and there are plenty of people about. Some say hello, others don't. No one stares, though.

Evan is now back at the hospital and I am at home, exhausted.

2 September 2013

Leaving the ward today feels strange. When I arrive there in the morning there are so many people standing around, waiting to say goodbye. I'm not at all sad that Evan and I are leaving, of course, but there isn't the same feeling of 'escape' I experienced when we left the ICU or Blythedale. Everyone at Yorkhill has seemed to be on our side throughout Evan's stay here, even when they didn't agree with me. And the standard of care has been much higher than in the US.

I feel apprehensive about the journey we are setting out on, and the challenges that lie ahead for Evan. But now we have carers in place, support systems and a real home and all of that allows optimism to grow. We have fought off so many negatives in our journey together, and now we can live in positivity. That makes things so much easier.

Eventually, with supplies packed up and farewells bid, I roll

Evan out of Yorkhill, into a taxi and, finally, bring him home, as I always promised him I would.

3 September 2013

This morning, on his second birthday, Evan Louis Schwarz wakes up in his own bed in our home. We have a music session at TouchBase and he wears his new superhero sweater. He is fawned over by everyone (and of course, I herald his birthday everywhere we go). Then, this afternoon, we go for a walk in Newlands Park in the sunshine. When we get home we have a mini concert with a tambourine and some drums. Then we have birthday cake with his granny. It's night-time now and he is comfortably tucked up in his own bed in our home.

I'm not sure there has ever been a better two-year-old's birthday.

22 September 2013

THE SCHWARZ FAMILY REUNION!

This weekend is our first ever Schwarz Family Reunion. There are thirty-something Schwarz cousins scattered all around the world. A while ago a few of them had the idea of having a reunion here in Glasgow, where all our parents were born and grew up. Madeleine couldn't make it, unfortunately, as she has taken up a new assignment to work in Nairobi and couldn't get the time off.

I Believe in Evan

On Friday night we host an evening in our house for the early arrivals to Glasgow. Evan sits with us and listens as tales of myth and misadventure from our childhoods are unravelled. When his carer arrives at 10pm, I take him off upstairs and we get him settled. When I come back down, I realise the folly of allowing Mum to sit with three infamous female cousins – they have plied her with wine and the effects are showing. When the rest of them go off out for an Indian meal, I am left to guide her into her room. It's one thing dealing with someone who is not at all used to the effects of alcohol, but it's another when you have to coordinate their movements with a walking stick and general immobility. Rounding her bed is the most problematic and she becomes a little stuck – with a leg either side of its corner – for quite a few moments. Once safely on top of her bed, the room starts spinning for her. She is fine the next day, although I certainly don't let her forget about it.

On Saturday morning about twelve of us cousins and Evan take part in a sponsored walk organised by Yorkhill hospital as a fundraiser. We start at the hospital car park, make our way to the Riverside Museum and the Tall Ship on the River Clyde. Then we walk along the river walkway, past buskers and artists and a service in remembrance of the Spanish Civil War (there's a statue of La Pasionaria on the walkway). When we reach the High Street we cross the river and head south into the Gorbals, then into the East End, past the brewery and back to the North Side across a little bridge over the Clyde, with rowers and canoeists passing underneath. We arrive finally, having walked five miles, at Glasgow Green. After congratulating ourselves and receiving our medals, most of the cousins go off to the pub to find the rest of the reunion party. Evan and I come home for a well-deserved rest (five miles feels a lot further when you have a buggy, a child, a pulse-ox, suction bag and a heavy vent to push around).

In the evening we go back out again, this time with all of the cousins for the weekend's big event at a nearby hotel. Evan is beautifully dressed in a woollen cardigan and denims. Mum drinks water. Photograph after photograph is taken, mostly with Evan in the middle.

Family life, it feels, is finally normalising in its own sweet way.

6 October 2013

We're really getting our money's worth out of TouchBase (actually, it costs hardly any money at all). Susanne has shown me all sorts of techniques for playing with Evan. Everything has to have a sensory purpose of some sort. For touch, we mix cornflour and water into 'gloop' and push Evan's hands right through the chalky mess so that he can feel the resistance and then the release at the end. We also put his hands into a bowl of dried lentils (we've dried the gloop off first) so that he can get the sensation of them falling away or slipping through his fists. Another trick is to use shaving foam. That's the easiest actually as Evan gets a wash in the process, even if he ends up smelling manlier than a two-year-old boy usually would.

Evan's interest maintains throughout and every now and then we get to see a finger or a foot twitching or a little movement from his wrists in response.

I Believe in Evan

Usually we have music playing, but we also have some games centering around certain songs. We have a drum log now — it's about three feet long and a foot wide and is a hollow log with slats in the top. Depending on where you bang the beater a different note will sound. Because of its size, I can sit Evan on top of it and hold him with one hand while I beat the slats around his bottom with the other. He can feel the vibrations and, hopefully, start to learn to hear the sounds too. I've got a range of other percussion instruments, like bongo drums, that I tap his little fists against, a couple of maracas and a selection of tambourines. For the most part, Evan's eyes remain wide and almost curious throughout the music sessions we have.

For help with vision we use lights. Violet sent Evan some birthday money and we used it to get a black tent, which sits in the peach room at the front of the house. I crawl into it with Evan and let all sorts of lights shine. Different colours bounce off the black walls, and magic wands glow green. Every now and then I am rewarded with an eye movement. Often, though, the light show proves to be quite tiring and he falls asleep.

Susanne has introduced me to the idea of giving Evan little mouthfuls of yogurt or jelly to inspire his taste buds, as the only other food he receives goes directly into his stomach through his feeding tube and never meets his mouth at all. He gets just enough of a mouthful to cover the front half of his tongue. Then I massage it around his mouth a bit with my finger. Sometimes I can feel his tongue pushing back in response.

We don't do a lot with smell. It seems to be the hardest sense to try and stimulate for Evan. Because the vent provides him with air through his tracheostomy, he doesn't ever breathe in through his nose, and so the usual mechanism for experiencing smells isn't there any more. We try giving him little whiffs of perfume samples from magazines and department stores, but it doesn't seem to have any effect at all.

The best thing about Susanne is that Evan clearly loves her. She is gentle and quite quiet, which, even before Evan became ill, is exactly what he is like. When she arrives you can almost see him slipping on to the same wavelength as her. In one visit recently, as Susanne was getting ready to leave, Evan actually raised his left shoulder up, asking for a cuddle from her. She was visibly touched.

It was a beautiful moment.

27 October 2013

I'm taking a break from organising Evan's Halloween costume. He's going to be a Blues Brother (I think every American male has dressed up as a Blues Brother at least once in his life, so this is Evan's turn). He will be wearing a white shirt and black tie, a black trilby hat and, best of all, will have an inflatable saxophone around his neck. The saxophone is supposed to hide his vent attachment, but it doesn't really. I can't wait.

Evan has only been home for two months, but I can't imagine a time when he wasn't living here. We have reached a wonderful level of comfort. I am around him all the time: in the morning, throughout the day, and when he wakes up in the evening. He always has his mum close by.

I Believe in Evan

I take Evan out a lot now. I've mastered getting him (and all his equipment) in and out of the car. I have also entirely overcome any concerns I had about the public's reaction to him. I suppose, initially, I was terrified that he wouldn't be accepted in the way any other little boy would. It reminded me of my own years of worrying about rejection when I came out of the closet. I have come to realise that, although I am entirely positive with Evan when we are among people who love us, I have at times been guilty of 'seeking disapproval' from strangers.

Once you give off that sort of vibe, disapproval is all you are going to divine from even the most innocuous of reactions. Overnight, I converted my own 'outdoors' outlook to the same positivity I have for Evan indoors, and the difference has been absolute.

Putting out the vibe that I am proud of my son and that I adore him is all I need to do, and every single reaction to him ever since has been kind and friendly. Just the other day we were in a tea room at the Botanic Gardens and an elderly man who was just leaving came up and gave Evan a little wave and made a funny face for him. Interactions like this happen all the time now. I love showing my little boy wonder off to the world, and in return the world shows its love for him. I call it 'The Evan Effect'.

We have been spending a lot of time at Sense's TouchBase centre in Kinning Park. It can be a stressful experience for Evan when he is taken out of the car. It takes a few minutes to get his buggy organised with the vent, before he is lifted out of his car seat and into it. Then it all has to be checked to make sure he is safe. It's always cold and windy at the front door of the centre, for some reason. Evan puts on his grumpy face. This is quite a feat since his face still doesn't move. He becomes teary and he gets a very angry look in his eyes. He sinks his chin down into his chest (although the trachy and vent circuit get in the way). His skin goes red and blotchy. For a boy without use of any of his facial muscles, no speech and minimal voluntary movement ability, he has found a way to make his opinion known. Once we get inside though, and he realises he is at TouchBase, the tears go and his face looks calm again. His eyes look happy – he loves it there.

We get a music lesson on Tuesdays. Jo Jo, Evan's teacher, lets him lie on top of one of the big drums, or on a blanket on the ground beside the piano pedals. When she starts playing either of them he can feel the vibrations. You can see he is concentrating on what he is experiencing.

On Fridays we go to TouchBase's sensory room. It's much bigger and better than the one at Yorkhill. Evan sits and stares as the colours change in the plastic tubes filled with water and bubbles, or watches kaleidoscopic images projected onto the walls. Susanne and I sit and chat as I hold him. I like to think Evan feels secure, listening to both our voices.

Often, when we get him ready to leave TouchBase, he puts on his grumpy face again, but he usually relaxes once the car starts moving.

We still get visits at home too. Susanne comes once a week and has new ideas every time I see her.

All of this has led to more improvements in his movement

and extra little phonating sounds and – the biggest news of all – he is breathing! A week or so into being at home, I realised he was taking a lot of his own breaths in the evening. I tentatively took the vent off and sat with one hand on his chest (to make sure it was rising and falling properly) and the other on the Ambu bag (in case his sats dropped). The first few times of seeing him breath off the vent reminded me of the first few times I ever went 'no hands' on my bicycle as a child. Exciting, daring, amazing! Since then we have been building up his time off the vent very slowly. Right now he can manage an hour every evening. When his heart rate starts to increase on the pulse-ox I know he is working too hard and I put him back on the ventilator.

I have a different reaction to all of these improvements than I would have done had they come along in the early days. Instead of feeling high as a kite and rushing off to tell someone (only to be shot down) I now sit and wait to see if it happens again, and then again, and then again. Then I wait for someone else, like a carer or someone at Sense, to notice too.

I used to pray for an overnight recovery for Evan. I know it won't happen that way but I also know that the patience I've learnt is invaluable. And it's starting to pay dividends.

I myself am doing pretty well too. Gone is the fogginess I always felt when Evan was in hospital. My mind feels sharper now. I put that down to a generally improved state of happiness. I have started attending a Master's course in law advocacy at Strathclyde University, in the centre of Glasgow. It's condensed into five intense weekends over the course of the year, and so far it's worked well, with carers covering extra shifts to look after Evan when I am there. It's a start. I'm really enjoying it.

I'm still very much enjoying living with Mum, too. Every night when the carers arrive at 10pm, and after Evan is settled upstairs, she and I sit and watch TV downstairs and make each other laugh. At some point she nods off and I have to wake her up to tell her to take her sleeping tablet.

I'm baking a lot of bread (nothing left to decorate) and it's very therapeutic. I have quite a nice life right now, all things considered.

Things are working out really well with the carers. Usually we only get one carer per shift, but the coordinating team know that I would always prefer an extra person on with Evan, and if there are any without an assignment, they double up with our carers. They are all very professional but also very easy to talk to. And they all adore Evan. He likes them too, although he hates getting dressed in the morning (his stiff arms always pose a problem). Often I get up to find him beautifully washed and dressed but with a grumpy look on his face. A cuddle from his mum soon sorts that out, though.

When there are two carers on overnight, often they go the extra step of washing Evan's hair in the morning. They inflate a plastic basin-type bowl with a hose that allows excess water to drain into the sink next to his bed. Then they wash his lovely light brown curls and give his head a good massage. I can always tell when they have done this. Aside from the fact that his hair gets lovely and soft and smells nice, he also looks as relaxed and content as it is possible for any child to look.

I Believe in Evan

In the evenings and for most of the day on weekends, there are no carers: it's just Evan, Mum and me. Those are the very best of times. I have all my people with me, in the same house, and often in the same room. I feel entirely safe. Mum and I often remark on what a happy home we live in. She loves having Evan here. Often she says out of the blue, 'Oh, Evan, the love that you are and the love that you bring to this house!'

I still get down days, of course. A few weeks ago I thought briefly of not believing any more, of assuming this is as good as it gets. I know I could cope with that, because I know I will cope with anything for Evan. I lasted a day and a half with that mindset and then I gave in. I missed hope, I missed optimism. I think everyone has to have that in their lives.

Most days though, I believe in a better tomorrow for Evan. At any rate, I believe that he and I will continue to be happy together. Will that be because I become entirely accepting of the condition he's in? Or because he will one day learn to blink and to breathe all the time and maybe even to walk and talk? Could I ever get to listen to his loud and breath-fuelled attempts at whispering as I've heard from other children? Or even just see him smile again?

I don't know what our future holds. Then again, I never did. I couldn't see one day ahead on 16 February 2012, so I can't pretend I can see five, ten, fifteen years down the line. And, because I don't know, I can afford to keep hope in my heart. I might get a miracle, I may get to keep the balance that Evan and I have right now, or things could take a turn for the worse.

So now, on good days I stare into Evan's eyes and believe one day his face will burst into a smile. His arms will flap around and his little chubby hands will grab onto my hair. His legs will find life and he will kick me in the boobs. On bad days, well, I try to remember there's a good day around the corner.

Who knows what challenges lie ahead.

When love is the answer, the question is bearable, whatever it may be.

17 November 2013

Evan has a play-date this weekend. My friend from law school, Mariya, comes up from London with the older of her two boys, Caspar, aged three. Evan and I meet them off the train at Glasgow Central and all four of us go for a walk around the Christmas stalls in St Enoch Square. From there, we go window shopping up and down Buchanan Street. It is still warm enough to sit outside so we have pizza at the terraced tables at Royal Exchange Square. Caspar has met Evan before, at Evan's christening, and isn't at all confused or phased by the machines or by my suctioning of bubbles from Evan's nose and mouth.

Now that we can get out and about, I'm rediscovering Glasgow. It really is a beautiful city. When the sun comes out, it can be quite spectacular. It rains a fair amount, but nowhere near as much as it is reputed to. And when the rain stops and the sun comes out again, everything looks sparkly. The greenery and the buildings and the windows all stand out then. The wet roads reflect the newly blue skies and the tarmac turns into a beautiful midnight blue. It's Glasgow's hidden talent.

When Evan, Mariya, Caspar and I arrive home, we fire up the chimenea and sit in the garden, watching the flames. Evan's supplies come in cardboard boxes. Sometimes there are so many of them I have to make two car journeys to get them home. The recycling bin can't take all of it, so I have started breaking the boxes down and burning them in the chimenea. The lovely smoky smell fills the house and drifts upwards to Evan's room. Perhaps he can smell it. At any rate, it's a relaxing thing to do. Sometimes watching those boxes burn, knowing everything is under control, smelling the fresh smoke in the cold air, all feels a little magical.

31 December 2013

I hardly write at all any more. In the early days I wrote almost constantly. My diaries are full of words engraved onto page after page of angst. Some pages even have holes where I pressed too deeply – too full of despair. I'm content enough now not to feel the need to write much, I suppose. I feel at ease with life now that Evan is home. I love all our activities. We are out most days, doing something he enjoys, and that something is almost always at TouchBase.

I also love our evenings together when the carers are gone. Evan and I sit and cuddle endlessly. I tell him how much I love him. Sometimes I tell him I am sorry this has happened to him; other times I tell him how lucky I feel to be his mum. Almost every night I tell him that he and I are in this together, and that no matter what, 'I will get you "there", wherever "there" may be.'

At Home

There is a song that is current right now by the band, Mumford & Sons. It's called 'I Will Wait For You'. Quite often I play it to him. When it finishes, I tell him that I will wait for him. However long it takes, however much help he needs, I will always be by his side – I will never give up on him.

He still gets an evening massage. Afterwards, when he's in his pyjamas, at around eight every evening I put him in his big beanbag chair and sling the vent across the back of it. Then I wheel him into the kitchen, where I cook dinner. Whether or not he can smell the aromas, he's lovely company.

I honestly cannot say I am unhappy any more, not at all. My life is full of love for Evan and hope for his future.

And Evan continues to improve. He has had so many little movements of his feet and hands. He has even managed to give a couple of voluntary bangs of his drum. That was big news! His eyes get brighter every day. He can move them a little more now than before. I'm hoping one day all of his little improvements will start happening at the same time as each other, and that his development will take off from there.

We have a new addition to the family: his name is Rocky. He is a black collie cross and he is ten years old. I got him from the pound on Thanksgiving. He is very gentle around Mum, ignores Evan until someone he doesn't know gets too close (in which case he either barks or pushes himself between them), and he can play rough and tumble with me. He suits our home perfectly.

TouchBase is still as good for Evan as it has ever been. We discovered in music class that a ukulele is a perfect fit to lie against Evan's body while holding him and playing it. It means he can feel the vibrations. I bought myself a purple one and am taking lessons. Our favourite tune is 'Twinkle Twinkle Little Star'. When it asks, 'How I wonder what you are?' I always ad lib, 'It's just gases' – no need to keep Evan in the dark.

We have also started going to art classes at TouchBase on Wednesdays. That means we get to go to the centre three times a week now – I'd go every day if we could. Imelda, the art teacher, starts the lesson by running one of her long dreadlocks through Evan's hands so that he knows who she is – this is called her 'signifier'. (Susanne's signifier is a little ceramic rose that Evan gets to hold, and Jo Jo sings a special song ('Hello, Evan') when it's her turn). Imelda then runs all sorts of different textured fabrics through Evan's hands. Some are soaked in paint, or water. Then she gets him to help her mould them into shapes, using her hands over his. The end result is always something quite spectacular: a solar system with all the planets in order hanging from string. A bowl covered in paper. At our last session before Christmas, Evan left festooned with all the decorations she had helped him make. A tangerine decorated with cloves, wrapped in ribbon to be hung from the tree. An ornament made from the unravelled spiral wires of an old calendar, with silver foil balls and white ribbon. I hung that on our front door and it looks amazing. 'Evan made that,' I tell everyone, with huge pride. We have stars and a wreath too, but the wire ornament is my favourite.

A week before Christmas we went to the Christmas carol service at TouchBase. Mum came too, with her friend

Kathleen. The music therapists all played lovely music, some of the admin staff got up and sang a few songs too, but best of all, so many of the children took to the stage and sang or read a poem. A couple of times, children would launch themselves on to the stage uninvited and would have to be coaxed off so the next act could come on. One little girl was in the middle of an impromptu version of 'Away In A Manger' when a staff member tried to stop her. It was far too adorable though, so the crowd booed and cheered until she was allowed to stay and complete the song. Another little girl swooped on our table and lifted the last piece of cake. Her mother grabbed her too late and was mortified. We, of course, didn't mind in the slightest. After a couple of hours Evan began to get a bit grumpy and antsy-looking, so we had to leave. I could have stayed all night though, it was that good.

Mind you, Evan's Christmas contribution to Sense was pretty good too. Susanne asked me a couple of months earlier if Evan could be the poster child for Sense Scotland's annual Christmas Appeal. I said of course he could! We got some pictures taken of him doing all his favourite things at TouchBase, and a flier was made with the caption 'Twinkle Twinkle Little Star' (coincidentally). The text was a letter from me, explaining how Evan and I had had a very difficult time but now we were in Glasgow and going to TouchBase things were getting so much better. It asked people to give money to support Sense. If people wanted to donate there was a little star on the flier that they could cut out and send a message alongside their cheque.

The staff have attached all the stars they have received to

pieces of string and wrapped them around four large pillars in the cafeteria. There must be hundreds of them, and many of them bear a special message for Evan. He and I walk around the pillars, looking at all the lovely things people say about him and about Sense and TouchBase. The appeal hasn't finished running yet, but it has already broken all prior records for Christmas donations.

That's my boy!

A few weeks after the flier went out, I got a call from someone at Sense asking me if I would do an interview with BBC Radio Scotland about Evan. I said I would so long as it got some publicity for Sense and TouchBase. We arranged that the interview would take place at the centre and when the day arrived, I took Evan along. It was a lovely experience. The interviewer was a lady called Mo and we talked for hours about Evan.

It aired just after midnight on Christmas day. You could hear the sound of the vent as I spoke, but you could also hear Evan's nice gurgling and phonating sounds too. I recorded and added it to a slideshow of pictures of Evan from the entire year and sent it to friends as our Christmas greeting to them. It's amazing to see how Evan has come on in these last twelve months in Glasgow. He's definitely bigger and now looks like a little boy. His eyes are wide open now and there is so much more expression in them. I'm in some of the pictures too. I don't know whether anyone would detect a change in me, but I can see that I too am doing better now than a year ago. This time last year we had just come home to Glasgow and everything was new. I was burnt out. I was scared and I lived with the most horrendous fear. Over these past twelve months I have gradually grown with Evan and now the fear I have is manageable. The hope I have for him is stronger than ever. And although I've never loved him anything other than with everything I have, because I feel so much better about him and our situation I can feel joy again as well as love.

6 January 2014

Score! Our general check-up with Dr Davies today, back at Yorkhill. There are six or so doctors in the room, as well as a couple of nurses. We go through how Evan has been: no infections, sats at 100 per cent with no added oxygen, time off the vent now, three hours at times. After all that, Dr Davies tells me that he is amazed that Evan is doing so well. He says again and again that it is incredible how far he has come, especially since he hasn't had to be admitted back to hospital once since he was discharged, which, apparently, is exceptional for any ventilated child. Dr Davies says that a large part of Evan's improvement must be to do with my insistence on getting him home. Then he adds, 'He has done so much better than I ever thought he could.'

'Well, I did tell you that he would,' I manage to reply, tears welling in my eyes.

13 January 2014

It was my birthday yesterday. Honestly, it was the best birthday ever. I didn't tell the carers because I knew they would offer to cover the weekend to give me time to myself. They've done that before, when they had extra staff on. One Saturday morning I found myself standing in the middle of Buchanan Street, with the rain coming down in sheets. I had no money, nothing to do and was missing Evan terribly. So I made sure that my birthday weekend would be preserved for Evan and me together.

It gets off to a great start. I meet my friends Emma and Rhonda the day before for a birthday lunch. Evan, of course, comes too. I love taking him out now. We have to rush home quite quickly as we stay out for so long the vent battery starts to run low, but we get home with plenty of time to change it. I have absolutely no issues with that vent now – I know it won't let us down, and since Evan can get off it for more than three hours at a time now, I really don't think he will need it for too much longer.

Yesterday, on my birthday proper, Mum agreed to come out for lunch. Evan and I take a taxi to Silverburn, an indoor shopping centre close to home. I have discovered that he loves it there – I think it's the smoothness of the ground as I roll him along, as well as the bright lights. He stares up at them, and always looks entirely content. Mum and her friend Kathleen meet us at the coffee shop and we have a lovely lunch. I can't get over how bright Evan's eyes are becoming. He still has the same limitations in body movement (i.e., hardly any movement at all) but his eyes are amazing now. We have a very enjoyable lunch and I am so proud to sit with my boy on my lap the entire time.

Later, as I roll him along to get a taxi home, an elderly gentleman stops to talk to us. He asks about the vent. I am happy to explain it to him. 'I have dementia,' he says, once I finish. He doesn't look ill – in fact he looks very healthy. It's not the first time Evan has attracted someone with ailments of their own, and another example of the Evan Effect. I like to think that because Evan and I are comfortable, it helps other people to share their issues with us. I tell the man I wish the very best for him. He gives Evan a smile and walks on.

Later, at home, I make a steak pie for us, and add pastry strips to it so it reads 'HB, 43, Me'. It's delicious, if I do say so myself.

Tonight, I am basking in the afterglow of a wonderful weekend with Evan. He and I are sitting on the couch in front of the fire. He is wearing his new pink and purple furry onesie and I have just played him 'Rainbow Connection' (by the Muppets) on the ukulele.

I'm still not very good, but Evan doesn't care. He loves it, and I love him.

22 January 2014

What an amazing night last night! Susanne from TouchBase invited us to a concert at the Glasgow Royal Concert Hall. Everyone in the audience was either disabled or someone's carer. Ten or so TouchBase children went, but there were people of all ages with all sorts of disabilities. Eight acts came onstage and sang a couple of songs each, all dedicated to us, the audience. I sit with Evan in my arms (although he is asleep for most of it). At the end, all the acts come back onstage together and sing 'Lean On Me' by Bill Withers for us. It's a wonderful experience. At the end, Evan, as usual, draws so many smiling faces over to us. He is a magnet for happiness.

5 February 2014

Mum's daily carer, Mary, has taken February off to go and see her new grandson in Australia. I have taken over looking after Mum. At first it was a bit difficult to juggle both Mum and Evan, but today I really think I've mastered it.

This morning I get up, change Evan's trach (with the carer's help), come downstairs and give Mum a shower, get her dressed and give her breakfast, take Rocky to the park, have a coffee with a neighbour on the way home, then get Evan ready and out of the house and into the car, and off to TouchBase for his art lesson.

Later, as Evan and I lie on the couch together, I can feel his little hands move in mine. It is as if he is saying, 'Well done, Mum, you're getting the hang of this.'

10 February 2014

Another great day at TouchBase today. When we arrive for music, Evan is really quite grumpy. It is very windy when I take him out of the car, and he hasn't quite realised that he is in his favourite place. When I take off his snowsuit, his sats start dipping. We manage to get him settled but I'm left feeling a bit stressed. Jo Jo decides to use the big orchestra drum. I hold Evan against the side of it with my left arm. Jo Jo starts playing notes on her cello, and I am given the big woolly beater to bang the drum with my right hand. It is a wonderful stress reliever, and it actually sounds really great too. Evan can feel both the vibration of the drum as well as the movement of my body each time I hit it. He looks quite amazed. His eyes are so bright – probably the brightest ever. After the lesson we stay for a coffee because he just looks so engaged. It's another wonderful day.

20 February 2014

I've been a bit low for a few days. It might be because we just had the two-year anniversary of Evan becoming ill. I can't quite put my finger on it, though. I've been feeling kind of… strange.

This afternoon we have a good visit from a visual aid specialist. We sit in the front room upstairs as she checks Evan's vision.

'He's definitely sensitive to light,' she says, as Evan's eyes draw towards the window when she re-opens the curtains. This cheers me up quite a bit.

Once she has gone, I hold Evan tight, telling him how much I love him, and that if I've been a bit unhappy for a day or two it isn't because of him.

Because with Evan in my arms everything is very, very good.

31 March 2014

Evan died on 21 February 2014. He was two and a half. It started with the hiccups, then his heart rate became very high. At 3am his carer Karen woke me up and told me he had a fever. We bundled him out into the car in his Gruffalo onesie and with all his equipment.

His death was as kind to both of us as it could possibly be. Our last day together was beautiful. Our favourite nurses were on duty and Evan must have felt me laughing with them as I held him in my arms. The lab results were all coming back negative for infection and it looked as though we wouldn't be in for long. We cuddled all day and when he slept in my arms I read a book. We had no idea what was to come.

I left at 6pm to get some sleep. At 7.30 the nurse called to tell me Evan's temperature was sky high. By the time I arrived back at the ward there were eight doctors and nurses around his bed, pumping fluids into new ports and holes made in his little body. I had to physically push away the nurses who were asking me to wait in the relatives' room. Standing at his head, while the doctors worked on his body, I kissed and stroked him and told him it was all okay, his mum was here now. Half an hour later, he was gone.

He died in the care of some of the best doctors in the country. As I watched them do compressions on his heart as it started to slow down, I knew – even though I didn't want to – that this was where the story ended. Later I learnt that Evan's brain stem had finally given in. That was why he could no longer control his heart rate or his temperature. Eventually, it was what left him unresponsive in his final hour. I have no doubt that nothing could have stopped him dying.

As I held him in my arms and felt the raging fever leave his body, two doctors consoled me. 'We always worried that this could happen,' one said. His tone was gentle and kindly. 'You know, we have all learnt an awful lot from your love and devotion to Evan. It has really been quite remarkable. Initially, we didn't think he would ever get to go home, but it was because of your love and perseverance that he could. And these last six months have been so good for him there. You can be very proud.'

The next week was a blur. Family and friends flew into Glasgow from wherever they were in the world. Anne and Pauline guided me through each day. Visitors arrived in an endless flow. Sometimes I could speak to them, but usually I couldn't. And yet I didn't want to be alone. As a compromise often I lay on my bed in the attic, listening to the chatter of familiar voices downstairs. It was the best I could do.

Evan's funeral was beautiful. The night before, we held a party at home to celebrate his life. Some friends gathered lights and lined the garden path from the gate to the front door with them – Evan loved lights. Jo Jo, his music teacher, came with her cello. Cousins and two friends of mine from childhood sang beautiful songs for him. I even sang the 'Evan Song'. The house was full of love for Evan – it was consoling.

When the next day came, I stood at the top of the attic stairs in my party dress (I'd asked for no black to be worn) as Pauline tried to coax me down.

'I'm scared,' I said.

'I know,' she replied.

I Believe in Evan

I sat with Evan's body for a last hour before it was time to go to the church. When the funeral directors arrived I knew everyone was worried about how I would react. 'Let's just do the very best job we can for Evan,' I told them. And we did.

When we arrived at the church it was packed. Angela B had arranged for brightly coloured balloons to welcome us at the entrance. A selection of important people in our lives, Anne and Pauline, Violet, Angela and Neil, Emma, Liz, Mariya and Margaret, formed a processional line and walked down the aisle, each with a bouquet of colourful flowers in their hands. They placed them on either side of the altar. The priest followed them, with his staff. Then came Evan and me. The two undertakers, strong in their softness, carried his coffin at either end, as I walked beside it, with my hand on it the whole way. In my other hand, I clutched a little posy of snowdrops a cousin had brought from her garden in England. At the altar, I lay the posy on top of Evan's coffin, then bent over it to kiss his name on the silver plate on top and to tell him, 'I love you.'

A family friend, Jacqueline, read the eulogy I had written. She did it perfectly.

We left the church as we had come in, with my hand on Evan's coffin once again. We emerged to sunshine and beautiful blue skies. 'He's brought the sun out for you,' said one of the undertakers.

Once I was back in the car with Evan's coffin, I sat and watched the mourners leave the church. Among them I saw Dr Davies. I got out of the car and ran over to him. I couldn't really speak, and he looked very emotional too. I managed to say 'Thank you' to him and we hugged.

Evan and I took our final journey together to the crematorium. Guests followed in a long line of cars, each with balloons tied to them. When we got there the priest said another few words and then Jo Jo and another music teacher from TouchBase, David, played 'Rainbow Connection', she on her cello, with David playing the banjo and singing.

It was pitch perfect in every way.

And now I grieve. It is a very simple grieving – simple inasmuch as I am capable of feeling happy for Evan. As I held his body after he passed away, I could feel the looseness in his limbs and I knew his brain had released its terrible grip on his muscles. It had also let go of the numbness of his face. He looked content, peaceful; there was even a hint of a smile. When I think of him in heaven, free from his machines, now able to run and laugh and jump and chatter, I know I couldn't possibly ask him to come back. I hope he is with Connie Connolly and with everyone else I have loved and lost. I hope he isn't missing me.

Now, as I dismantle the coping mechanisms I installed when Evan was alive, I wonder if I can ever rework the sum of all their parts to cope with life without him. People tell me no one can take this pain away from me. Sometimes that feels sympathetic, other times it feels like they're saying, 'and we're not even going to try.'

It hurts me beyond belief to think that people think of Evan and me with nothing but sadness now. How unfair. Evan is love.

But I am told I will never get over this loss. Apparently, there is no negotiation. I am now the ghost of Evan's mum. And I walk alone.

Every day has too many hours in it. There is too much time to think about my lost hopes, dashed dreams. There is a void in my heart that is bigger than me. And how can a void feel so heavy? I miss Evan terribly. I miss him in every word I speak. When I think of life in New York, I miss him. When I fill the car with petrol, I miss him. I miss him in the colour of my tea. There is nothing that doesn't make me think of him.

My constant fear is gone, manageable though it had come to be. It has left a hole that nothing better has filled. Grief comes in waves, crashing violently against my heart for the most part. Sometimes my head hurts so badly because I can't force enough tears out to satisfy the pain. At other times it feels like I cry so much I am turning into a liquid, ready to be brushed down a drain. Swoosh! I get so sad I can't focus my eyes, and I only realise when my vision becomes blurred. My heart feels like a steel rod has been forced through it like a thick skewer.

10 May 2014

Mood changes come hourly now, rather than minute by minute. I've learnt to stop trying to fight grief. I let it happen. It feels just as bad, but is slightly less exhausting. I don't fight the moments when I feel okay either, like I did in the beginning. Before, I felt I was being disloyal to Evan if I wasn't feeling total misery at all times. Sometimes now, when the waters lap the shore more gently, I can reach out to Evan and feel his love. There are times when I can feel him in my heart so strongly it is physical. It feels fit to burst.

I wonder about the dream I had, a year or two before Evan was born. I have no doubt even now that the young man I saw was Evan. And yet it didn't materialise. But I chose to believe the dream and not the doctors. And that decision was the first of many vitally good choices.

Evan and I lived his life with a lot more love than fear. It scares me now to think how suddenly he died. It had been mentioned to me that this could happen, but I ignored the possibility and chose to hope instead.

Hope allowed me to believe Evan would get better. It let me give him as much positivity in his life as I could. Hope got us through the ICU in New York City, resisting the pressures to 'withdraw care'. Hope kept me almost sane through our ten months at Blythedale. Hope got us on a plane to Glasgow, where our hearts and spirits flourished, even if Evan's brain did not. It was hope that brought him all the way home – really home – to his granny's house, where the three of us lived in love and a new kind of happiness for six whole months.

In Glasgow, our hope held a chorus. Nurses and carers, even a doctor, got behind us. The people at TouchBase supported us with their drums and cellos and with their flashing lights and laughter. Hope, in all these forms, lit Evan's road with light and allowed love to flow – to overflow, rushing, gushing.

And it wasn't just Evan's road, of course, that shone brightly.

Let's not forget the Evan Effect. That boy brought out the best in so many people. He brought love and joy; he raised people's spirits. He focused so many people on the importance of life and of love. He made me realise how much I want to live.

Of course, sometimes I feel so sad and sore that I think I really don't want to be alive right now. Violet tells me I have to stay alive because that's the only way to keep Evan in my heart. She tells me I have to let my heart mend because Evan needs to be able to live there. But there are times when I feel almost certain that I must follow Evan, that joining him in heaven is the only way through this pain. Sometimes I wonder if he needs me to be with him. Is he safe wherever he is? Is he missing me?

But the Catholic education so deeply engrained in me reminds me that I don't know for sure, if I take my own life, that I will be reunited with Evan. Perhaps instead I will buck a system that is patiently waiting to reunite us at the natural end of my time on earth. But if I wait, and suffer through life without Evan, will he still be in heaven by the time I get there? Or will his soul have been recycled back to earth and we will miss each other anyway? How does it work? And why don't we know? These are the kind of thoughts that keep me awake most nights.

A few days after Evan died I found myself in the garden, in an aimless, cloudy state of mind. I saw a little chestnut; its shell was nearby. There are no chestnut trees that I know of for at least a few blocks. Perhaps the wind carried it to me. It had a little red shoot coming out of it, and it had been trying to dig into the soil. I left it where it was. A week later, I found it again. Its shoot had grown, but it was still finding it difficult to get a hold in the soil. I picked it up and put it in a pot with some fresh soil and compost. The shoot is six inches long now. If it keeps going, I'll plant it in the front garden, to replace the smaller silver birch. We'll see.

The holly tree is still standing. It didn't fall down after all. Perhaps it would have preferred to, but it didn't. The remaining branches never expected to feel the elements – they always thought that they would be protected by higher ones, but those are gone now. This tree will never look the way it once did, tall and stunning. The stump will always be visible, but there is some new growth on the remaining branches. It looks like it will grow wider and fuller now, instead of taller. It will be different than it expected to be. It might even, eventually, be better.

19 July 2014

I've been trying to take baby steps forward. Not long after Evan died, I had to attend another university intensive weekend. I wasn't going to but the teachers were so kind and encouraging. 'It will get you out of the house,' said one. 'You don't have to participate if you don't want to,' said another, 'just come and be around people that really care about you.' So I gave it a go. The first of the three days was hard but people were nice. The second was impossible – I had to leave early. On my way home I stopped several times, sometimes to wretch, sometimes to sob uncontrollably. When I finally made it home I went straight to bed and wept and wept.

The third day we were to do a mock trial. The sleep had done me good and I felt much better, so I decided to take part. I wanted Evan to see me at my best, doing a good job, and making him proud of his mum. The room we used for the mock trial looked out on to a patch of grass. When I wasn't advocating as best I could, I concentrated on that patch of grass, imagining Evan rolling and jumping and laughing all over it.

'Absolutely excellent' was the critique I was given.

'There you go, Evan,' I told my son. 'That's for you.'

My little boy in heaven can still inspire me.

After that, a couple of things fell into place and just yesterday I had a meeting in Edinburgh. The journey from home to Glasgow Queen Street railway station was daunting. The suit I wore was a couple of years out of style, and my larger waistline was certainly giving it a run for its money. More than that, though, I haven't felt normal in such a long time. Going out in public is especially challenging. I see Evan's shape and size in every brown-haired boy I pass (and there seems to be no other type of child any more). Everything new I do is a challenge these days.

As I walked into Queen Street station I suddenly thought of Evan. It was startling. I saw him in his brown Gruffalo onesie, with his big blue eyes shining bright. More than a thought, it was incredibly intense. I had to take a moment to the side of the station entrance, crying behind my sunglasses. Once I composed myself I found my train and made my way to Edinburgh. The meeting went really well. As I left the office and walked across the Royal Mile back to Waverley train station in the scorching afternoon sun, I felt it again: Evan was right there with me, in his woolly onesie. At first I worried he was too hot. Then I realised this wasn't a thought: it was that other thing. It was the presence of the spirit that so many people who have lost someone they love will tell you they experience.

I have felt Evan many times since he passed, but not to that extent. A little baby's frame nestled into my side as I sat down for my first grief-counselling session. One afternoon I was awakened from a nap by the touch of a child's finger poking my left eyelid. When I woke there was no one there. Imaginary hands have touched my back as I've felt little hugs from Evan. Photographs of him randomly pop up on my phone and computer. Other little hints of his presence appear here and there.

Last night I kept waking to the sound of Mum's radio downstairs – she lets it play all through the night. Around the third or fourth time I realised it was the same song that was playing each time I woke. It was Mumford & Sons, 'I Will Wait For You'.

And this, I like to believe, is my cue. I am challenged to suffer and manage this pain and work my way through my own life as best I can. I have to accept that life is about getting through. It's about loving with all of your might, and feeling the agony when the person you love goes. It's about taking tiny steps when you want to take big ones. It's about falling over when you want to stand on your own two feet. It's about feeling defeated and down and dusted. And then it's about feeling the love of the people who care about you, the kindness of those who ache only slightly less than you do but hide it to protect you. It's about the people who will do anything to make things just a little easier for you. It's about the tiny building blocks that one day make you realise you feel a little stronger than before. And those moments when, suddenly, you feel a little bit of optimism. It's about looking back and knowing you have loved, fully, wholesomely, absolutely. It's about knowing that, no matter how painful, it was all worth it.

So I will live through this pain, and one day I will live as happily and as well as I can. And at the end, I will meet Evan in heaven. In the meantime, I will always hold Evan in my heart. I will never give up on him. I will never stop believing in him.

Epilogue

I cry less, these days, but grief still has a way of sneaking up on me and knocking me sideways. I can look at Evan's baby pictures now, the ones from when he was well. I can see his gorgeous smile. Those pictures almost always make me happy. I can't yet look at more recent ones, but I will, one day. I'm sure of it.

Six weeks after Evan died, my Irish friends sent me a ticket to Mayo on the west coast of Ireland. We laughed and we cried, and we walked for hours across the rugged landscape, between mountains and lochs and oceans. They handed me an envelope. There was a generous amount of money in it. I'm going to use it for some kind of memorial to Evan. I've been thinking of a bench in the park, with a little plaque with his name on it. It should say something like, 'When you sit here don't be sad, just think of the love my mum and I had'. Perhaps the Evan Effect can continue to soothe.

Already there are several memorials for Evan. His carers brought plants for our garden, and a couple of friends gave me young trees and seedlings to plant in his memory.

One time, when Emma was visiting, I reflected on how I brought Evan home from New York. 'No, he brought you home,' Emma corrected me. She is right: I am where I need to be. I am being very well looked after. I miss being the one doing the caring, but I have to forgo that role for now. Even Mum is more use to me than I am to her at the moment.

I have been thinking a lot about the pain of grieving. It is not correct to say that 'no one can take away your pain', and perhaps I was giving too literal a meaning to the phrase when I started to hear it so often in recent months.

The fact is that yes, they can take it away. Not directly, of course, but tiny piece by tiny piece. Pain is a big brick wall, blocking my light. It is dark and terrifying. Sometimes I thrash and flail against the wall. Other times I slump down onto it, giving in to its misery and sadness. Sometimes I believe I have to get used to the darkness and other times I just can't bear it. But sometimes, often really, people come and take away a brick here and there and let some light in.

Emma and Rhonda always seem to show up at exactly the right time with a plate of food or a bag of logs. (I spend hours staring into the flames of the chimenea in the back garden.) Other friends arrive unannounced to walk the dog or bring groceries – they all let a little bit of light in.

The Irish trip, of course, helped, as much for the comfort of companionship as the change of scene.

Epilogue

My friend Brian, back in New York, told me that he ran a half marathon with the stub of a football game he and I had attended in his pocket the whole time, in tribute to Evan and me. That removed a brick or two. Letters and emails sending love, the cards from strangers I have received over these past few years, they all remove bricks, whether at the time I receive them or when I read them again later.

Friends who have lost children of their own remove many bricks. Casper's mum, Mariya, who lost her first child at birth, invited me to her home in London for a weekend. Her husband, Tim, took their two children away to a friend's so as not to upset me, which was as thoughtful as could be. Seeing how Mariya and Tim have managed to build a happy family if not in spite of their loss, then definitely because of it, gave me the first insight into how things can eventually become okay.

Kevin, my friend since infancy, who lost his daughter at seven and a half months, reminded me of how strength rebuilds and eventually, at least sometimes, the goodness that comes from your child's life makes up for the heartache of losing them. And perhaps inadvertently he gave me an outlet for those inevitable moments when the wrong thing was said by those meaning only to help. 'Scrambled eggs,' he explained. 'I was so fragile that they could well have been saying "scrambled eggs" to me and I would have dissolved into tears.' So now, when I hear someone say something that could cut me in two, I try to think of scrambled eggs instead.

For those realities that are too painful to observe right now, such as little children playing in the swimming pool or at the park, I have my friend Debbie, in Florida. She lost her husband several years ago and knows only too well that the most innocuous things can cut like a knife at times of great loss. She invited me to email her a rant anytime I feel like it. We usually end up laughing at how insensitive some people can be when they've never worn the crown of pain, like we do.

Anne comes to visit as often as possible. Whatever my mood when she arrives, by the time she leaves, she has always removed a dozen or so bricks. Pauline calls frequently. She visited recently with her children, who don't remove bricks so much as brush them effortlessly aside as if they were never there in the first place.

A surprising source of light came in an email exchange with an ex-girlfriend. She only heard of Evan's passing quite a few months afterwards. We hadn't been in touch for years, and had parted on not-so-pleasant terms. In the course of the exchange she sent me this:

'You know what else makes so much sense – I was just thinking on a run – that this little boy Evan, with all his struggles, is only placed here for a short while – and who does he get for a mother? Of course, one of the people with the best ability to love here on earth. He doesn't get some crap mother, some selfish mother, some never-there mother – he gets you! I mean, it made so much sense to me. So that with the short amount of time he had here, he gets someone who showers him with love and made his journey here the best it can be.'

Brick, after brick, after brick. As I see it, when the bricks disappear, a beautiful beach comes into view. There is a new dawn emerging on the horizon and the cloudless sky is tinged faintly with pink and yellow. The water has a slight ripple but

Epilogue

other than that the waves are only gentle. Their rhythm is soft and soothing. There's a pleasant breeze. It carries the faintest smell of salt water and the freshness of the day. There are no distractions; everything is calm. I know Evan is not there, but I know that when I can be on this beach he will be everywhere. And that is when everything becomes okay.

In my heart, in my head, and on my beach, I will always believe in Evan.

Acknowledgements

First of all, thank you for reading this book. Any good in it flows directly through my lovely muse, Evan Louis Schwarz. All of its imperfections are mine alone.

There are many people – some of whom appear in this book and some who don't – who I will never be able to thank enough. In fact, I have so many people to thank that I'm worried I will miss someone. If I do, it's most certainly not from lack of gratitude. Here goes…

The Fire Department of New York (FDNY) paramedics who got Evan to hospital (on several occasions), saving his life each time.

Most of the doctors, nurses and other staff members at Columbia Hospital. I am truly grateful, even if the stresses of our month in your ICU unit did not allow me to show it at the time. There are a few people from our time there whose full names

I'm not sure of but who I want to thank individually. Joel the young minister who has wisdom beyond his years. Music Therapy Kate, who brings far more good to her patients and their families than I think I was able to encapsulate in this book. Soulemar the social worker, thanks for being on our side. Dr Baird and Dr Patrick (whose last name I didn't catch) were standouts amongst the medical staff, in a good way. Dr Jocelyn Brown was a fair and compassionate representative of her office and I thank her very much for respecting Evan and me as she did.

The doctors and nurses, therapists, assistants, vent technicians, security staff, and cafeteria staff at Blythedale hospital, where we lived for nine months. In particular, Evan's first schoolteacher, Angela Redd, and my pal, Andrea, a nursing assistant.

The New York nurses who assisted us during our two weeks at home. The nurse who accompanied us to Scotland asked not to be named, but she knows who she is and I am so grateful for her excellent professionalism. Kudos to the staff of United Airlines, who really were exceptional.

My siblings, Anton Schwarz, Anne Schwarz, Frances Sinclair and Pauline Schwarz all did their very best for their nephew and their sister. I am so grateful that they were around to help, whether it was to visit, to call or text, to pray, or just to make sure mum was okay too. As Pauline says, 'We may not always be close, but we always pull together in a crisis.'

Kathleen Gilbride, Mary Reilly and Margaret McNulty removed additional weight from my shoulders by making sure Mum was well cared for during this time (and still do). Mum's carers at Cordia also helped out a great deal.

Acknowledgements

Of course, the trauma of our hospital experiences in New York was cushioned over and over again by the love and support of many wonderful people who I'm so lucky to call my friends. Deborah Donenfeld was first on the scene and remained an incredible source of support throughout our ten months in hospitals. Jackie Frank – oh Jackie Frank – what a powerhouse of love and support and practical solutions and lifts to and from hospitals and courthouses! Jackie mobilised and encouraged many more members of our networking group – BNI Chapter 12 Manhattan (The Flagship Chapter) – to come and visit and I doubt I would have survived that first month without that level of support. Rebecca Klinger, a frequent visitor, provided Evan with relaxing massages (and taught me how, so I could give him massages in Glasgow). Stacey Francis, another frequent visitor, did everything she could to ensure I was financially protected, (and also makes a mean devilled egg).

Liz Duwe – what a friend. I guess she was undeterred by my manic complaining on all those evenings in Valhalla Crossing and the Cabin. She is an incredible source of love and support and everyone should have a friend like her. Same goes for Brian Kluepfel, who was a very entertaining source of distraction when needed, and another shoulder to cry on. Neil Schreffler, Esq., my law mentor, provided important legal advice and also helped me to gain a perspective on some of the doctors, based on his many years handling medical malpractice cases. That was invaluable. And he made me laugh a lot too.

Randi L. Karmel, Esq. is a wonderful attorney and a very dear friend. I've represented friends before, and I know all about the sleepless nights that go with that territory. I especially wouldn't want to have me as a client – not in this particular situation anyway. But Randi did an incredible job under tough circumstances. She is an excellent lawyer, although I hope you never need to use her services.

Violet Lennon, Evan's godmother and my wonderful friend, has been a source of love and strength and support on an incredibly consistent basis, despite living in another country throughout. I know how strongly she still holds Evan in her heart and I love her for that.

Clare Grill was another standout supporter and visited us on a frequent basis. Like Liz Duwe, she spent long days with Evan when I could not. This gave me incredible comfort. After Evan died she sent me a drawing she had done of two birds, and a note that said it reminded her of Evan and me. Every time I look at it I think of her and I think of Evan and I know exactly what she means.

Other friends from our stateside experience that deserve special mention include, Gail Frank, Ilana, Sean Lundy, Brenda Tunney (who brought lots of lovely meals to the hospital for us), Gerry Sugrue, Edel Durack, Mariya Talib, Angela and Neil Bryson, Myko Winiarski, Stephanie Del Marco, and Anne Chenebenoit, who brought me that first notepad and told me to 'write it all down'.

Melina Diaz brought work documents and mail to me from the office we shared, allowing me to serve out my clients as best I could. Jayson Grimsley frequently fixed my computer for me (for free), which was my lifeline to the world at times.

Debra O'Donnell was a wonderful therapist. I should also,

Acknowledgements

though, give thanks to my original therapist, Jennifer McCarroll, PhD, who set me up with many coping mechanisms that have come in very useful in these past few years.

The staff and management at 160 w.71st Street, New York, NY 10023 outperformed. They treated us with kindness and compassion and provided all sorts of help. They really broke the mould of the New York Landlord.

My clients, who I wish I could have continued to represent. Thank you for being so understanding.

Yorkhill Hospital has since been shut down and a new children's hospital has now opened as a wing of the Southern General Hospital on the south side of Glasgow. Yorkhill may have been the hospital Evan died in, but it was also a place he lived in for many months too. Despite the end, and some of the scarier moments, I have nothing but gratitude and respect for the doctors, nurses, and assistants there. (I hope Dr Phil Davies comes across as the thoughtful, caring and intelligent doctor that he is.) The family care services at Yorkhill were far superior to any other hospital we experienced. The chaplaincy visitors were always a welcome sight; the social services department helped me greatly in finding out my rights when I returned to Glasgow; even the clown doctors weren't that scary once you got used to them. And the music lessons from Julia – again, a service that is invaluable to the morale of any children's hospital ward.

I can't say enough good things about the ventilation team in Glasgow. Elspeth Jardine, Helen Grier, Morag Anderson, and Claire Goodfellow all run an exceptional service. Each of them are incredibly personable and they always made me feel that they were going above and beyond for Evan and me. Evan's carers — what love they showed him. Louise, Julie, Morag, Nathalie (and I know I've missed a couple more names but I'm truly grateful for what you all did for us) and especially Karen. It was because of Karen's experience and professionalism that Evan was taken to hospital, where he died in the safest of circumstances, and in a manner that gave me no need to wonder if there was anything more that could have been done.

Sense Scotland's Touchbase centre at Kinning Park, Glasgow. Oh how I love Sense! JoJo Landers and her beautiful cello, Imelda and her wacky artistry, Mháiri Doherty, Alison Sommerville, Rachael Tonge, David McLuskey, the staff at the front desk and behind the lunch counter, the fundraisers, the admin people — all of you brought an incredible amount of joy to Evan and to me and I will never think of you with anything other than warmth and happiness. And of course Susanne McLean, a relentless source of inspiration to me and education to Evan. She's a mum herself now, I've been told, to two very lucky twin girls.

My cousin, Stephen Travers provided his hotel, Number Ten, on the south side of Glasgow for Evan's christening, which is a day I remember with great fondness. He also raised funds for Yorkhill in Evan's name, and found ways for me to do the same. For Evan's celebration party he provided food and drinks for the guests.

The Schwarz cousins rallied throughout to support us. I'm not going to name all thirty-something, but I do want to highlight Pat Woods, Con and Peter Reilly, Catherine Mulvey, Alexandra Murdoch, Michele Schwarz, and Madeleine Schwarz.

Father Michael Woodford of St Gabriel's Church, Merrylee

is a wonderful man and priest. He was a source of joy at Evan's christening and a source of comfort around the time of his funeral. Anderson Maguire, the funeral directors, provided us with a wonderfully dignified and beautiful funeral. And they didn't even charge us for it. As mum always says, 'Make sure you use them for mine!'

Jacqueline Gilbrook delivered the eulogy I had written for Evan. I still don't know how she managed to do it so smoothly and calmly and with such love shining through. I could never have managed it.

JoJo Landers and David McLuskey made me smile when they started performing 'Rainbow Connection' at Evan's cremation service. Special thanks to Dr Angela Dunn, Margaret McNulty, Emma Nicholson and Rhonda Chambers who rallied and continue to rally around through the grief.

I know there are lots of people who I don't know or who I barely know who sent prayers and good thoughts to Evan and me throughout our journey and I am very grateful and very touched that they took the time to think of us.

The faculty and students at the LLM Advocacy course at the University of Strathclyde – and especially Dame Elish Angiolini, QC and Gillian More – provided a good distraction and lots of hankies. I also learned a lot about writing that I hope I've put to good use in this book. Thanks to them for their kindness and their patience.

Having taught me to read and write, Pat Schwarz has always been my *de facto* editor. But of course, I could not have poured much of the nightmare onto these pages if I thought my mum would read it. So she and I have agreed this is a book she will never get her hands on. That takes nothing at all from the fact that she is a wonderful mother, and has been just a star throughout all of this. I'm glad she is Evan's grandmother, and I am very proud she is my mum.

In Mum's editorial absence, Violet Lennon has been my go-to person from the earliest drafts right through to the end. She has a great eye for an error, and a wonderful knack of saying what works and what doesn't work without inflicting offence.

Mariya Talib, Barbara Richards, and Alison Sommerville (Alison works at Sense Scotland) each read early drafts and provided really valuable insights and suggestions. Brian Kluepfel and Liz Duwe read an almost final draft although both cried too much and forgot to give me suggestions. Still, it was nice of them. Alexandra Murdoch, Michelle Schwarz, and Madeleine Schwarz also read drafts and sent their love and encouragement too.

My agent, Robert Dudley, was kind enough to take me on. He's a very good guy. He has always left me with the impression that this is a project that is personal to him. My editors, Anna Marx and Chris Mitchell, have been a delight to work with and I'm grateful to them and everyone at John Blake Publishing for their care in publishing this book.

Finally, as you might imagine, I have left the best to the end. My greatest love and deepest gratitude go to my darling son, Evan. The boy who brought out the very best in everyone, especially me. No matter the heartache and pain – and there has been lots of both – the love this boy has given me, and the love I have for him far outweighs it all. Evan, I would go through it all again – all of it – for the joy of your life, in mine.

I love you.

Appendix One

Letter to Norma

Norma,

I write this letter to you under two assumptions.

The first is that you shook my little five-and-a-half-month old baby Evan. Since every doctor that has ever looked at his medical notes has concluded that he was definitely shaken, at least twice, since only you and I were alone with him (at separate times) and as I know for sure that I did not, and could not ever have harmed him, then I have to believe them.

The second assumption is that you didn't do it deliberately. It hurts me far too much to think of you or anyone hurting Evan so I have to believe this too.

I have replayed those months again and again in my head.

The first time Evan went to hospital they should have done a CT scan. But they didn't. I took him to his doctor after he got home and the doctor said everything was fine. A few days later, when you videoed what you thought was Evan having a seizure, we went back to the doctor and showed it to him. He said it wasn't a seizure. As I found out much later, he was wrong – so wrong. We were relieved, though. I believe – sincerely – that when Evan had more seizures you panicked and shook him to try and get him out of them. This was an incredibly stupid reaction. In fact, it ruined our lives.

You are not the sole culprit, of course. We relied on two different doctors. They were at fault in not doing their jobs properly. I take responsibility for my lack of intuition. I will never stop wishing I had known better.

In the early days after the massive brain haemorrhage Evan suffered, I felt concern for you, no matter what the circumstances. Then I felt anger. When the ACS case was brought against me and not you, I felt even angrier but I found a way to let it go. I realised that I could only help Evan if I was 100 per cent positive. Feeling anger wouldn't work. I suppose I also felt that it couldn't be true. I didn't believe the doctors any more by then, so I felt able to think you hadn't done anything but love him. That changed when I finally worked out that your statement to ACS had been full of lies.

All of this is what leads me to my theory that you were stupid and careless, but that you weren't trying to hurt Evan.

Appendix One

I don't think the police will ever get their act together to even so much as question you. Also, if my theory is correct, I'm not sure that there's much point in you going to prison. Whatever the truth is, though, none of it will help Evan.

I am taking this opportunity to lay out in full everything I want to say to you: to tell you how much your stupidity has hurt Evan's life and my life.

As you know, the last time you shook Evan he suffered a massive brain bleed and cardiac arrest. That was the day our happy lives were torn apart. We spent a month in ICU. I was told there, first that he wouldn't live, then that he was so badly injured I should withdraw care: let him die. I refused. Thankfully he survived that first month, but he had to have a tracheotomy operation (because he can no longer breathe on his own, he needs to be ventilated 24/7) and a tube inserted into his stomach through which he was fed. Then we moved to a rehab hospital, Blythedale, in Westchester. At that stage, he was still deeply comatose. He didn't open his eyes for three months. When he did, they were lifeless. It took at least eleven months from when you shook him for me to really feel that he was no longer in the coma.

As I write this, Evan is still fully ventilator dependent, still gets fed through the tube in his stomach, and still has almost no ability to make voluntary movements.

His face is numbed – that's the best way I can describe it. Nothing works. His eyes open, but he can't blink. He can't fully close them either. This means that I have to tape his eyes shut when he is asleep to protect them from drying out. His mouth can do nothing: he can't smile. He can't move his tongue or close his mouth. When he tries to cry, his face doesn't move. All that happens is that he gets very red around his eyes and tears roll down his still cheeks. Soundless.

The brain bleed left him with high tone. This means his shoulders and arms are very tight – they sometimes refer to it as spasticity. I don't know if he would be able to move his arms if that weren't a problem, but I do know that simple tasks, such as being dressed in the morning, can become extremely painful for him.

I know when he feels pain because I can see his increased heart rate on the monitor that has been attached to him since the last time you looked after him. As a matter of fact, other than his silent tears, that is almost the only indicator I have of how he is doing. If his heart rate is high, I know something is wrong. If it is low, I know he is calm and comfortable.

The ventilator keeps him breathing, but there have been many times when he has come close to dying anyway. Sometimes he gets a mucous plug in his trachea. If I can suction it out through his tracheostomy tube he will be okay, but if I can't, I have to do an emergency tube change. I suppose I'm just about used to that now, but there have been some extremely scary moments in these last eighteen months.

Appendix One

I try and stay positive, and don't listen to what the doctors say. If I listened to them, I don't think either Evan or I would still be around.

I do know, however, that, if things stay as they are (and they have pretty much stayed the same for eighteen months), Evan will never be able to walk or talk or have any real ability to function in life at all.

I also know that I have missed out on all the wonderful events that these last eighteen months would have brought to our lives. His first steps, first words, the sight of him running to me for a cuddle – I don't know if I will ever see any of that now.

What makes all of this bearable, of course, is how much I love him.

There have been many other effects on our lives too. I stayed with Evan throughout these past eighteen months and gave up everything that might be a distraction. The first casualty of that was my law practice. I had spent five years building that practice and I loved it but I had no choice but to give it up. Money became very tight (I had no income for a long time, and the disability payments I eventually received didn't cover everything), so I had to sell the house that I had in Brooklyn. Later, I had to cash in my pension. I don't have any of that left – it all went on getting through these last eighteen months.

I had to get a new apartment (the rehab hospital told me they wouldn't send Evan home to me if we still lived in the studio apartment). That was very costly, but I had to do it.

I Believe in Evan

As Evan's discharge date came closer, though, it became obvious to me that I couldn't stay in New York. My memories of the two hospitalisations of Evan when he was in your care haunted me so much that it became unbearable to live at the same location. Also, I needed the support of my family. Although I had wonderful friends, New York had become an increasingly lonely place to be. I decided to move Evan back to Scotland, where I am from. That meant breaking my lease and losing my security deposit, as well as paying the expense of travelling (we had to hire a nurse to come on the flight with us) and moving our belongings over to Scotland, too.

Evan has spent the last ten months in hospital in Scotland. He is going to come home, finally, next week. That will be just in time for his second birthday. He and I will be living with my mother in her house: I don't have any other place to live and no money anyway.

I honestly believe I have forgiven you for what you did to Evan. That is not out of any sense of righteousness, it has always been a protective mechanism that came naturally to me. I knew from the very beginning that I had to keep all my good energy flowing towards Evan to help him. I simply couldn't afford to focus on you.

There have been times, though, in the depths of my grief that I have felt overwhelming hatred for you. For all those days where I simply couldn't cope with what had happened to Evan, thankfully, there were also one or two good days when I could feel calm and hopeful. In those times I realised that my hatred for you was valueless.

At other times of great stress – taking Evan out for the first few times, with all his equipment, preparing for the daunting journey back to Scotland with him – I thought of you with anger. But once we got through and over these difficulties, I remembered, once again, that having negative feelings about you just doesn't do me any good.

All of these effects of your actions aside, there is, of course, the issue of the family court case that ACS brought. You allowed me to go through that without ever raising your hand and admitting that it was you, not me, who had shaken Evan.

You let them drag me away from Evan's bedside and down to court where I had to watch, helpless and sobbing, as they removed Evan from my legal custody. You let them put me through six months of hell. Even when your name was added to the petition and you were accused alongside me, you didn't own up. When a medical expert wrote a report saying that, because of the timing of onset of Evan's cardiac arrest and brain haemorrhage, and the fact that you were the only one with him during that time and for eight hours prior, you had your lawyer argue technicalities.

As well as doing nothing to help the truth be known, you also lied. You lied about where you had been that day, about how Evan was doing and about what he had eaten. When I asked you directly what had happened – and told you Evan's treatment might depend upon your answer – you still lied and said nothing.

I can understand you were scared, but did you feel any

concern about how scared I was? About Evan's future, our lives together, and about whether I would lose custody of him because you wouldn't own up?

When push came to shove and you knew you couldn't win against ACS, you surrendered to the court's jurisdiction. This was cowardly. It means that you didn't have to say what you did to Evan; you just had to take the punishment. Really, though, there wasn't much punishment for you at all: three months of supervision, counselling, and not being able to work with children again for twenty-eight years. When you look at Evan's life and my life now, and all the things he and I will never be able to do, I think you have to admit you got off very lightly.

Once the ACS case was over, things got slightly better for me. Although it cost me a huge amount of money to defend, at least the lawyer's bills stopped increasing. The constant stress that I was under eased a bit and I felt a lot less anxious. I suppose at the same time, you finally sank back into irrelevance in our lives.

Until very recently I truly believed that, as the victims, Evan and I had to focus on our own healing, and that I could trust the New York Police Department to take care of getting justice for us. It's unlikely now, as I said, that they are going to do anything. I have come to accept that I can't afford to care. It's something I can't change.

Also, though, I don't need to think about you serving out twenty years or so in a state prison in New York and all the suffering that would bring to your own family. What I need – all I have ever needed – is to be allowed to focus on making Evan's life as happy and as positive as possible.

There are certainly still times that I feel I can't cope with this situation, times when the restrictions on both our lives feel overwhelming. But those times have become less and less frequent.

I can't speak for Evan, but I know that, if I had to choose between being in your position or being in mine, I would choose to be Evan's mother every time. But I also know that no matter how difficult my life has become it is bearable. Most importantly, I love Evan with all my heart and would do anything for him. There are times that I genuinely feel quite sorry for you.

Sincerely,

Elise Schwarz

Appendix Two

Evan's Eulogy

Oh my darling Evan,

I am so sad, my wee honey boy, not to hold you in my arms again. But I hold you now, as I always have and always will, so deeply and so strongly in my heart. Our golden bond of love won't break.

Our first five and a half months were wonderful together. Oh, such joy. Then we had nine months of fear and sadness and pain, but we still had love. And cuddles – lots of them, all day, every day. And then we came to Glasgow and we were wrapped in the love of our friends and family. Strangers too.

We had nine months in Yorkhill, where you were adored

by the staff. You and I sat in our corner together for hours on end, reading, stretching. Then the sun came out and how it shone for you all summer long. We got out almost every day, for a walk or home to Granny's beautiful garden.

In these last six months when you came home to live in Granny's house with me, we found a new level of happiness. Every day you made me feel like singing to you. Every day we cuddled with love and fondness for hours. Your carers loved you too, but they had to do the things that made you grumpy – like getting you washed and dressed – ha ha. We found Sense Scotland in Kinning Park and they shared our hopes. They gave us a place to learn and listen and see lights and hear the most beautiful music. And they allowed me to protect all my hope that you would get better. That made all the difference to us both.

I always believed that you would get better. I am so glad of that. It allowed me to give you everything, without holding anything back. I fought the doctors and I fought anyone who said you couldn't improve. With help from so many people, we kept your life as positive as could be. And you did improve. Your eyes grew bright, you started breathing again on your own: you did your very best. Your doctor told us just a few weeks ago that he was amazed at how far you had come. As you might recall, I took great pleasure in telling him, 'I told you so.' And as I've always told you, Evan, your mum is never wrong. Right now you are running and jumping in heaven, flashing that gorgeous broad smile of yours, and laughing your hearty little chuckle. We did it, Evan, we won. We are the champions, my son.

Still, it's hard for me to imagine that you are gone now, and I know I am not alone in sometimes questioning God's decision to take you. But God has blessed me with love for you and kept me mostly free from anger during these past two years and so I owe it to Him, but also to you, to find the good in your passing for those of us still here on earth.

Two years ago I was told you might die within hours. If you had, it would have been such a painful tragedy, so hard to understand. But here we are, two years later. It's painful, but it has so much meaning.

In your entire life, Evan, you have never done anything wrong. Your whole life has been love, and you have brought so much love and sincerity to everyone I know. Your big cousin Catherine reminded me that in these last few years we have lost three cousins, an uncle, my dad and her mum Kate. During all that time of sorrow, you have been a beacon of love, binding our family closer than it has ever been.

And the love you have brought to me, of course. I don't know why I got so lucky, but God chose you and I to do this together. He chose us to love each other, and he chose us to remind the world of what love can do.

I loved you from the moment I held you, and I will never stop loving you. I am so grateful for the purity of that love. It has guided me since you were born and even now you have died, it will guide me to you for as long as I live. What a blessing.

I Believe in Evan

Whatever my life has been or will be, Evan, you are the shining star in it.

I know you can see me crying, and perhaps you are asking why. And so many people are crying for you. We must be sad. We must miss you and wonder how to get through life until we can meet again. But, my little darling, please don't confuse our sadness for despair. We can see the beauty of your life: your dignity and courage and, most of all, your love.

As I held you, after you had passed, a doctor came by to talk to me. He told me that he had learnt so much from my love and devotion to you. Well, he only learned half a lesson, Evan, because my love and devotion come from your love to me and from your beautiful spirit – it would have shone bright on a grown man ten times your size. He was nice, though – the doctor.

They all did their very best. But you and I both know that this was your time to go up to heaven. You will be so happy there. If you think you were loved here on earth, just wait till you meet your granddad, Uncle Lew, your Aunt Connie, and the rest of the gang. And Connie Connolly – she looked after me when I was wee – she will warm your socks by the fire and teach you all the songs I tried to play you on the ukulele. I know you will be loved.

But don't forget your mum. I love you more, and most.